Journey into Day

Journey into Day

Meditations for New Cancer Patients

Rusty Freeman

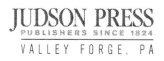

JUDSON PRESS
PUBLISHERS SINCE 1824
VALLEY FORGE, PA

Bible quotations in this volume are from the *Contemporary English Version* (CEV) © 1995 American Bible Society; the HOLY BIBLE: *New International Version* (NIV) copyright © 1973, 1978, 1984, used by permission of Zondervan Bible Publishers; the *Good News Bible*, the Bible in Today's English Version (GNB), copyright © American Bible Society, 1976, used by permission; and *The Living Bible* (TLB), copyright © 1971, used by permission of Tyndale House Publishers, Inc., Wheaton, IL 60189, all rights reserved.

Permission to reprint Robert Schuller's "The Hour of Power" (on page 42) granted by Crystal Cathedral Ministries. All rights reserved.
Permission to reprint text from Bill Hybels's *Honest to God* (on page 65) granted by Zondervan Publishing House. Text © Copyright 1990 by Bill Hybels.
Permission to reprint Tim Hansel's *You Gotta Keep Dancin'* (on page 85) granted by Cook Communications Ministries. © 1996 by Cook Communications Ministries. May not be further reproduced. All rights reserved.

Library of Congress Cataloging-in-Publication Data

Freeman, Rusty.
     Journey into day : meditations for new cancer patients / Rusty Freeman.
        p. cm.
     ISBN 0-8170-1350-4 (pbk. : alk. paper)
  1.   Cancer—Patients—Prayer-books and devotions—English. I. Title.
BV4910.33.F74   2000
242'.4—dc21   99-047478

Printed in the U.S.A.

10 09 08 07

10 9 8 7 6 5 4

To my beloved wife, Debbie,
who saw me through some valley-of-the-shadow nights

Contents

Introduction

THROUGH MY OWN EXPERIENCE, I learned that almost every single day of being a cancer patient has its own new and unique challenges. It is like being on a roller-coaster ride designed to upset our equilibrium at every turn. After having ridden the ride twice, I would like to help you make it through whatever particular turn, dip, or loop that today offers you with as much grace, faith, and sanity as possible.

Life is not designed with many inherent guarantees. "Death and taxes" is the old saying. The Bible adds a couple more—trials and the love of God. No human can guarantee anyone any more than today. So I would like to help you with today, whether you are facing a fresh diagnosis, a surgery, prolonged and painful chemotherapy, or even the struggles of remission. Everyone's ride is a little different, but there are some common twists and turns.

Some of the worst things about cancer are the new, unfamiliar experiences. When we run into the unknown, our imaginations can go wild. Several weeks into my first chemotherapy treatment I had an experience during which I thought I was dying. It was so frightening that I also thought I was having a nervous breakdown. My doctor explained that I was not dying; I had had a drug reaction. A Christian counselor explained that I was not having a nervous breakdown; I was scared. These calming voices helped me. Please allow me to be that voice for you.

Today you are walking through the valley of the shadow of cancer. But it is a journey into day because God is with you. God promises to bring you safely to the other side, to a place of green meadows, whether earthly or heavenly. Therefore, live in hope and fear no evil. My thoughts and prayers are with you until you reach the light.

Cancer Is So Limited

Cancer is so limited . . .
It cannot cripple love.
It cannot shatter hope.
It cannot corrode faith.
It cannot eat away peace.
It cannot destroy confidence.
It cannot kill friendship.

Cancer is so limited . . .
It cannot shut out memories.
It cannot silence courage.
It cannot invade the soul.
It cannot reduce eternal life.
It cannot quench the spirit.
It cannot lessen the power of the resurrection.

—Source unknown

The Collision

You're cruising down the highway of life, windows down, hair blowing, radio cranked up, enjoying the scenery. The pedal is down, and the engine is purring. All is good with the world. Suddenly, out of nowhere, it appears. At first it doesn't look like you're going to hit it. And then you realize it's in your path. You zig this way and that, trying to avoid it, but with one final, eye-opening revelation, you know there will be impact, and your survival is no longer in your control. You close your eyes and grip the steering wheel. "I'm sorry, but the tests are conclusive. You have cancer." Crash.

Life blindsides us sometimes. And there is no preparation for catastrophe. It's no good walking through life expecting someone to drive through every red light and smash into us. That wouldn't prepare us; it would only drive us nuts. We should live with a certain sense of indestructibility. Otherwise we would never enjoy the good times. But the reality is that life can be fragile and is always at some juncture terminal. Don't blame yourself for enjoying the good times. Give yourself some adjustment time to deal with the present circumstances. It's always a bit of a shock to be in an accident.

Dear God, calm me in my surprise.
Steady me while I find my equilibrium.
I thank you for being the link between
my ideal world and the real world. Amen.

Everything Has Its Time

Everything on earth
has its own time
        and its own season.
There is a time
for birth and death,
        planting and reaping,
for killing and healing,
        destroying and building,
for crying and laughing,
        weeping and dancing,
for throwing stones
and gathering stones,
        embracing and parting.
There is a time
for finding and losing,
        keeping and giving,
for tearing and sewing,
        listening and speaking.

There is also a time
for love and hate,
      for war and peace.

—Ecclesiastes 3:1-8, CEV

Giver of life, our time here is not one happy, straight road
but a ride down an untamed river.
Thank you that you take the trip with us. We are safe
with an all-knowing, all-caring guide. Amen.

Assuming the Worst

For many people, the very word *cancer* is synonymous with "I am going to suffer terribly and then die." Although that does happen in some cases, let me say emphatically that you could survive cancer, even with little discomfort. When you speak of cancer, there are many different kinds of cancer with many degrees of severity and various stages in a particular cancer's growth. A cancer that is caught early can be much easier to treat than a cancer that is discovered late. Sometimes it can be a veritable walk in the park. Some treatments are much kinder than others, and different people respond to the same procedures with an amazing degree of variety.

Sometimes a quick surgery or a little radiation will do the trick. A friend of mine, just diagnosed with prostate cancer, was all gloom and doom. He was contemplating doing nothing and letting the cancer run its course because he had watched his grown daughter die a long and painful death from breast cancer fifteen years earlier. "What did the doctors suggest?" I asked. "Thirty days of radiation," he replied. I assured him how easy that would be and that thirty days would be over before he knew it.

Two months later, after minor discomfort, his cancer was arrested, and he was going about his life.

Don't expect the worst. Your brush with cancer might not be any worse than having your tonsils removed.

Heavenly Father, worry is a monster
that eats up our lives. Give me peace as I wait.
I choose, in you, to hope for the best. Amen.

Your Oncologist

One of my oncologists explained chemotherapy something like this: We are going to put cell-killing drugs into your body. They cannot distinguish between good and bad cells, so they will destroy good and necessary functions as well as the bad and destructive. My job is to monitor your body's response so that we don't end up killing you in the attempt to kill the cancer cells.

Because of the nature of this fine balancing act, my first rule in finding an oncologist is this: He or she must be someone whom I trust is vitally interested in keeping me alive! This is neither the time nor place for half-heartedness.

Cancer treatment is often harsh, painful, and dangerous—be it an operation, radiation, chemotherapy, or a bone marrow transplant. There can be numerous and exotic side effects. I need to be able to look my doctor in the eye and say, "Do whatever you have to do to get me to healing or remission. Operate on me, radiate me, make me sicker than a dog for six months or a year, lock me up in a sterile room and destroy all the bone marrow in my body." To do that, I must trust that he or she will take care of the precious cargo that I am.

A good oncologist is someone who cares enough to have a system that responds to your needs when you have them. It is not necessary that you be able to speak to your doctor personally twenty-four hours a day, seven days a week, but it is necessary that he or she has a good network of partners, receptionists, and nurses so that you aren't ever left on your own. It is not necessary for them to win the warm-personality-of-the-year award, but it is necessary that they are dedicated and caring enough to make sure you get all the help you need whenever you need it. Take time to shop for an oncologist. Ask friends and neighbors which oncologists they were pleased with and which ones to avoid.

Father, thank you for the gifted and dedicated people who give their lives to save the lives of people like me. Lead me to the right doctor for me. Amen.

Feelings

Why don't I feel anything? It's been a week since the doctor said the C word. Why no tears, no terror? Why aren't I falling apart?

Now it is just a word that I'm dealing with. Soon I will be dealing with whatever punctures and jabs and surgeries and drugs that my case requires—but now I have only a word. It's not a nice word, and I've been pondering the implications of what the reality behind that word will do to my life. But it's still a vague and fuzzy word.

Numbness is a grief reaction. You are leaving the world (though you never really lived in it) of things being logical. Feelings, or a lack of them, are not dictated by the laws of logic. They often have their own set of norms that defy logic. Learn to stop saying, "How I'm feeling doesn't make any sense." It makes good sense, but emotion sense, not logic sense. Grief is not logical, but it does follow a pattern. Even at that, psychologists tell us that grief follows an individual pattern. Take some time to read about and to learn to accept and value your feelings.

Creator, you have made me much more complex
than I realized. I confess the mystery of my own self.
Help me to understand how you have wired
this marvel that I am. Amen.

God, Our Protector

Whoever goes to the LORD for safety,
whoever remains under the
     protection of the Almighty,
can say to him,
      "You are my defender and protector.
      You are my God; in you I trust."
He will keep you safe from all hidden dangers
     and from all deadly diseases.
He will cover you with his wings;
     you will be safe in his care;
     his faithfulness will protect and defend you.
You need not fear any dangers at night
     or sudden attacks during the day
     or the plagues that strike in the dark
     or the evils that kill in the daylight.

—Psalm 91:1-6, GNB

God, my defender,
I lean on you
Your strength holds firm
no matter how heavily
I ask you to shoulder the weight.
Cover me with your care. Amen.

The Bible

The Bible is God's eternal Word for the ages. It is also one of the ways that God communicates intimately with us through the Holy Spirit. Millions have experienced, as they were reading through its pages, a word or a sentence or a paragraph or a psalm that jumped out at them as if God were speaking to them and to them only.

Each time that I had cancer I found a certain Scripture that grabbed me and took on great significance. I would read that same Scripture almost daily, and each time it would minister life to my soul, give me hope, help me carry on.

God is. God is alive. God cares for us. In a mysterious process that I don't comprehend, God makes words that were written thousands of years ago become his private communication to me, his promise. Seek that word. Find that promise. Plant its seed in your heart. Let it be the rock that you hold onto when all else turns to Jell-O.

Living God, speak,
for your servant listens.
Give me a word of hope
to hold onto through the trials.
By your Spirit
turn ancient words
into a personal word for me. Amen.

Honest Communication

There is the temptation to try to protect people, to try to shield them from some aspect of the truth. This leads to secrets, loneliness, and mistrust. Most people function best if they feel that they are on the team. The team I am referring to are the people—doctors, relatives, friends, and neighbors—who are doing whatever they can to help you get through this crisis. Don't deprive them of the right they have to be concerned for you—to expend love on you. Besides, you need them. The Bible says that it is not good for humans to be alone. You need their cards and their prayers, the meals they drop off or a financial gift, their wisdom and their ears when you need to talk about some hard things.

I learned about honest communication the hard way. When I was first diagnosed with Hodgkin's disease, my wife and I had the usual black feelings that the word *cancer* conjures up, but we were void of information about what was ahead. Secretly, I hunted up what were at the time modern brochures. It said that my disease was about 85 percent curable. I thought, that means that there is a 15 percent chance I won't be alive next year. I didn't want to upset my wife, so I kept the information to myself.

My wife secretly looked up Hodgkin's in a 1950s edition of a home medical journal. It said that Hodgkin's was 100 percent fatal. She didn't want to upset me, so she kept this information to herself. Can you imagine our lonely suffering as we tried to protect each other? It was several days before we got together and started working as a team.

Dearest Friend, thank you for the other dear friends
you have given me. Together we will attack
this problem. I will cherish your gift of others.
Help me to lean on them as I lean on you. Amen.

Statistics

Statistics are the triumph of the quantitative method, and the quantitative method is the victory of sterility and death.

—Hilaire Belloc

It is our duty as physicians to estimate probabilities and to discipline expectations; but leading away from probabilities there are paths of possibility, toward which it is also our duty to hold aloft the light, and the name of that light is hope.

—Karl Menninger in
*The Vital Balance: The Life Process
in Mental Health and Illness*

Participate in the world of professional medicine, but don't sacrifice to it as a god. "You have such-and-such percent chance of survival." What does that mean? It sounds scientific. It means that of all the various people who have had this disease this percent beat the cancer. But it means little to the unique individual that you are. Even if there is a one in a million survival rate, how do you know that you are not that one? Even if there is a 100 percent mortality rate, that only means that all the people who have had the disease so far have died. It is no guarantee that you will. With life the saying holds true, "The surest road to failure is not to try at all."

With you, nothing is impossible, O God.
If you have it in mind for me to live, I will live.
In the meantime, I am alive.
While I am alive, I will choose to live. Amen.

A Prayer for God's Protection

I run to you, LORD,
for protection.
       Don't disappoint me.
You do what is right,
       so come to my rescue.
Listen to my prayer
       and keep me safe.
Be my mighty rock, the place
where I can always run
       for protection.
Save me by your command!
You are my mighty rock
       and my fortress.

Come and save me, LORD God,
from vicious and cruel
       and brutal enemies!

I depend on you,
and I have trusted you
  since I was young.
I have relied on you
  from the day I was born.
You brought me safely
through birth,
  and I always praise you.

   —Psalm 71:1-6, CEV

Mighty Rock, shield me from the windstorms of life
that seek to blow me away. I hear them howl
on the other side of your wall. I am safe in you. Amen.

Hair

It's such a small thing. Unimportant really. I should be thankful if it's all I have to worry about. And yet . . . Let me say first of all that not everyone loses hair. My hair remained on my head during my first year of chemotherapy. I was surprised. I had even bought an expensive hair prosthesis. But I was not so lucky the second time. About two weeks into chemo my hair all fell out in about a twenty-four-hour period.

I expected that it would happen, yet it was hard when it did. In this day when people shave their heads for a lark, what is so hard about losing our hair? First, it strikes our pride and our vanity. Many people choose to dye their hair purple and have it spiked. They seem to enjoy having people stare at them — and stare people do. But we have not been given that choice. It may not be in our nature to want people to stare at us. For us, it is like being forced to wear a clown's nose all day.

Second, hair loss is a daily reminder that we are sick. We get up in the morning, look at ourselves in the mirror, and know that we are fighting for our lives. Until our hair grows back (it normally does, though sometimes kinkier, finer, or thicker), we will not have the luxury of feeling normal or well. Everyone who looks at us will also be reminded that we are one of the walking wounded. The secret pity flows.

Try to put a healthy spin on your lack of hair. It's not there because the chemotherapy is working! The chemotherapy is killing cells in your body. Look at your bald head and say, "Die, you cancer cells, die!" It is also a reminder to your friends that you are going through a rough time. Be thankful when it spurs people to pour out love on you.

Finally, use your hair loss to bolster yourself like a soldier who has been scarred in battle. Lift your head with pride and declare yourself a veteran of life. Paul boasted that he had been knocked down but not knocked out!

O Lord, I know that you are concerned, not
about the outward appearance, but about the heart.
Help me to swallow my pride and receive
the good gifts that come with losing my hair.
Help me to be more than a conqueror. Amen.

The Unseen Barber

Swirling in the drain
clumps of hair
matted leeches clogging
the flow

my pride slips
away through
shower tears sprinkling
down.

Exposed scalp stares
in the mirror of my infant
self
regressing.

Tonight I will cry
my loss,
but tomorrow I shall wear
my nothingness
as a badge of
courage.

Father, I feel exposed
in more ways than one.
How quickly and easily
my hair fell out.
There was nothing I could do to stop it.
What else could happen
just as easily?
Protect me from unseen forces at work. Amen.

Rhythm

With some treatments this is not feasible, but if it is possible, find a rhythm to your life. Yes, some days are nightmarish, and our only goal is to get through them. And some days are a little less than nightmarish, but it still takes all the oomph we have just to lie in the bed and doze and daze the time away. But with some treatment cycles, there are good days and even great days! With some treatments, those days are even in the majority.

Try to find a flow to your life. Two days of hell, three days of vegetation, five days of good, and four days of great. On the days that are not so good, be at peace with that. Say to yourself, "Just another bad day or two and then things will get better." When the good days come, suck the marrow out of life. Enjoy them all you can. Dance with those endorphins as they bring healing to your body, mind, and soul.

Give me wisdom, Lord of life,
to see what you have set before me today.
Give me the strength to go when it's time to go
and peace to stay when it's time to stay.
I wait on your timing. Amen.

Job

Satan answered, "There's no pain like your own. People will do anything to stay alive. Try striking Job's own body with pain, and he will curse you to your face."

"All right!" the LORD replied. "Make Job suffer as much as you want, but just don't kill him." Satan left and caused painful sores to break out all over Job's body — from head to toe.

Then Job sat on the ash-heap to show his sorrow. And while he was scraping his sores with a broken piece of pottery, his wife asked, "Why do you still trust God? Why don't you curse him and die?"

Job replied, "Don't talk like a fool! If we accept blessings from God, we must accept trouble as well." In all that happened, Job never once said anything against God.

—Job 2:4-10, CEV

O God, I do not understand
why this disease has come upon me.
I know that pain and suffering
are sent by the devil.
Like Job,
I will keep trusting in you. Amen.

Lowering Expectations

There is an unloading that needs to take place. Consciously or not, we see ourselves as indispensable. The office will fall apart without me. No one else in the family knows how to cook. How will the children get to school in the right clothes? We'll end up in the poorhouse.

We need to see that a great deal of the problem is pride rather than survival. I talked with a straight-A student—in contention for valedictorian—who had a serious illness. She was agonizing over having to go to the hospital—"What about my classes?" she fretted. I smiled at her and said, "Jill, it's all right if you get a B. In the long run it won't matter much, but your health is all you've got. Why don't you give the other kids a chance to catch up a little?" She smiled and relaxed.

We do this in all sorts of areas. It's not that the kids won't eat; it's that they'll probably eat more junk food and frozen dinners than you'd like. That's okay. They'll make it on pizza and

McDonald's for a while. The kids will get to school dressed, maybe mismatched, but dressed. And the office will survive. You won't be the top producer this year, or you won't be able to do that expansion that you've been planning. While you have cancer, readjust your goals, expectations, aspirations. Say, "If we can get through this year in one piece, all alive, and not living on the street, we'll be doing well."

God, I confess that I'm the one putting pressure on me.
Everyone is giving me slack but myself.
Help me to let go and to concentrate
on what really counts. Amen.

Confusion

Has the bottom dropped out? Are you feeling panicky? All the formerly straight lines in your mind's house are all askew. All your formerly held beliefs and standards and practices are floating in a sea of uncertainty. Relax. Breathe deeply. These are temporary responses to all the new stimuli that your mind and body are experiencing. Besides simple shock and grief, confusion and agitation are side effects of some types of chemotherapy drugs.

I remember calling a minister friend with all these confused feelings. "I don't know if I believe in God anymore. Nothing makes sense. I try to read the Bible, and it sounds like gibberish." "That's okay," he said. "Don't worry about that right now. It will come back to you." He was right; it did. Chemotherapy drugs can have powerful effects on our mind and body. Learn to say to yourself, "It's just the drugs and the shock." Relax. Don't try to figure out the world right now. Wait until you are more clearheaded. It will be there. Give yourself the gift of not thinking about things that confuse you now.

> *Heavenly Father, I collapse in your arms.*
> *I surrender trying to figure out the world.*
> *Please, hold me and protect me*
> *while I'm weak and confused. Amen.*

Helplessness

Trusting a tenuous foothold
   too much
      high up in the branches
   of a magnolia tree
I fell
   in slow motion
      cartwheeling down
      being slapped by
   branches
       scraped and cut
falling
   pell-mell
      being tossed by
   unseen hands
      each obstacle
bruises rather than
      catches
       begins a new series
   of flailing gyrations
      when I reach for security it
      vanishes.

O Master, I feel so helpless,
as though there is nothing
to hold onto.
Please be there to catch me
at the bottom.
Help me to relax,
knowing that your strong arms are waiting. Amen.

A Prayer for Protection

I come to you, LORD,
for protection.
>   Don't let me be ashamed.
Do as you have promised
>   and rescue me.
Listen to my prayer
>   and hurry to save me.
Be my mighty rock
and the fortress
>   where I am safe.

You, LORD God,
are my mighty rock
>   and my fortress.
Lead me and guide me,
so that your name
>   will be honored.
Protect me from hidden traps
>   and keep me safe.

You are faithful,
and I trust you
because you rescued me.

— Psalm 31:1-5, CEV

*Satan, fear, danger, death, and disease attack me.
Protect me, God. Put your big arms around me
and hold me tight. I snuggle into your lap. Amen.*

Part of the Team

> On the other hand, it is all but certain
> that active participation in the treat-
> ment, were it only through laughter or
> the cultivation of the will to live . . .
> helps to mobilize the natural defense
> mechanisms of the patient which are
> the indispensable agents of recovery.
> —René Dubos in Norman Cousins's
> *Anatomy of an Illness* (22–23)

One of the worst things that you can do during
your treatment is to sit like a lump and let everything happen to you. Become a part of the healing team that is working on your recovery. Cancer
steals from you a sense of control. I felt that every
day of my life was a roller-coaster ride or reaction
to everything that was happening to me—unex-
pectedly getting sent for a CAT scan, blood tests,
trips to the emergency room, weeks spent in the

hospital, days spent too ill to care.

It helps to regain some sense of control if you come up with a game plan to help in your recovery. This doesn't have to be dramatic. Norman Cousins, in Anatomy of an Illness, tells how he designed his entire treatment. You can do much simpler things—but the point is, do something!

I came up with a low-impact exercise program, figuring that it had to be good to keep my blood moving. (Check this with your doctor. Remember, you're part of a team!) I would walk laps around the hospital corridors, dragging my IVs with me. I also did research on the best way to implement the diet I was on. It wasn't much, but I found out which of my favorite foods I could eat. This upped my happiness level. I also learned that humor was good for me, so I consciously made sure that I had some funny videos. Join the team. Work on your wellness.

Master, I will trust you. I will also do
what you have put in my power to do.
Show me the seeds of health. Amen.

Busy

I learned that a highly developed purpose and the will to live are among the
prime raw materials of human existence.
I became convinced that these materials
may well represent the most potent
force within human reach.

> —Norman Cousins in
> *Anatomy of an Illness* (71–72)

As best as you can, find something to be busy at
during your illness. Try not to sit around with heaps
of dead time and nothing to do but think about
how ill you are. Occupy yourself with something
that engages your mind and heart. Recent pain
research has even shown that by distracting ourselves we block the perception of pain in our minds.

One of my parishioners who has cancer has
poured herself into a backyard shrub and flower
garden. Cancer has left her blind. Nonetheless, on

her good days she feels her way out into her land-scaped garden and weeds and digs and plants. These days restore her soul.

Through both of my illnesses I continued on a part-time basis to preach and pastor. Helping other people kept my mind off of myself. Wisdom must be used in order not to cross the line of overdoing it, but to be doing is to be alive. Go to work if you can; immerse yourself in a hobby; give your brain something to feed on besides pity.

Master, you have given me gifts and talents
and interests. Give me the strength to keep going—
to engage in life. Block the pain with purpose. Amen.

Angry with God

"God is a big enough God to love you even when you're angry with him." Those were words said to me by a friend not too long after I had begun my first rounds of chemotherapy. I was hurting. I felt lost. I felt abandoned. I felt betrayed. Why would God allow this to happen to me? I was angry with God.

I shared my anger with a friend on the phone, and he said, "I believe that God is a big enough God to love you even when you're angry with him." It took having children for me to get the full impact of those words. Occasionally my children are in a bad mood; they're hurting, they're tired, they're frustrated, and because I am unable to make the situation better, they lash out at me, "I hate you, Daddy. You don't love me. You're a mean daddy."

I don't take it personally; my ego is not so fragile. I know it's the pain speaking. If anything, it makes me feel for them all the more. Are you angry with God? It's all right to express it. God understands. You are not committing some horrible sin. Like any good parent, God is a big enough God to love you even when you're angry with him.

Heavenly Father, I am angry with you.
I am confused and hurting. I know
that it is wrong to lash out at you—
at the same time that I am doing it.
Thank you that you don't reject me.
Thank you that you see past my outbursts. Amen.

God's Love

Can anything separate us
        from the love of Christ?
Can trouble, suffering, and hard times,
        or hunger and nakedness,
        or danger and death?

In everything we have won
        more than a victory
because of Christ who loves us.
I am sure that nothing
        can separate us
        from God's love—
not life or death,
        not angels or spirits,
        not the present or the future,
        and not powers above
        or powers below.

> Nothing in all creation
>   can separate us
> from God's love for us
>   in Christ Jesus our Lord!

—Romans 8:35,37-39, CEV

Dear God, whose name is love, I accept
the wonderful truth that I am the object
of your affections. And that, whoever on this earth
are the best examples of selfless love,
your love is more excellent. Amen.

Grief Process

One thing that happens to us when we hear that we have cancer is that something dies. What dies is our sense of invincibility. Even if we will eventually survive, we still have to begin to deal in a serious way with our own mortality. We begin to grieve the loss of ourselves as we are. One of the questions that may nag at us is if we are reacting normally. You may be acting quite normal, but it may be normal grief. Grief has its own rules of normalcy. When it comes to grief, there is a wide set of normal reactions.

Many people do not understand the grief process. The result is that they may accuse you of acting abnormally when you are acting as expected. They may create even more anxiety in you by questioning your mental stability.

Shock, denial, fainting, being speechless, and literally running away are all common ways people react to devastating news. Then there is the complication of trying to work through the grief process while you're going through staging and treatment. It is normal to have intense periods of grief with intermittent periods of relief. It is normal, contrary to popular belief, for grief to deepen, with no periods of relief, as with time the reality settles deeper into your psyche. It is normal for grief to take from six months to a couple of years. The intensity of grief will vary widely depending on personality and emotional maturity. Tears, anger, agitation, needing company, and wanting privacy are all normal reactions. As someone said, "Normal is only a setting on the dryer."

*God, help me to understand myself and to be gracious
to myself as you are gracious with me.
Help me in my grief, and lead me through it.
You know the frailty of my human makeup. Amen.*

The Mind

Pain is at least partially controllable by the mind. When I was a boy, there was nothing so dreadful to me as to have to go to the doctor and get a shot. Alarms would go off in my fight-or-flight system as soon as I learned of the proposed trip. By the time I was in the doctor's office, every fear button in my body was at red alert. Naturally, I fainted after each inoculation.

But through each of my cancer battles, I had to have a couple of hundred shots, IVs, blood draws. Little by little, I began to work on my attitude to shots. They hurt, but they weren't the end of the world. I found that if I consciously thought about it, I could make my body relax—that I could stand down from red alert to something close to at ease.

It is possible to force your mind to go to other places, to think about things other than the pain. Sometimes I could forget the pain by getting into a good, lighthearted conversation with the nurses or lab techs. Sometimes I would drift my mind off to an island in the Caribbean. I found that these techniques worked not only with shots but also for scans, chemotherapy injections, and even surgeries. Learn to use your mind to control your pain.

Master, you created me with sensors called pain to let me know there is something wrong in my body. Teach me, during treatment, to bypass some of those sensors, much as I turn off a car alarm. Thank you for this ability you've placed in my mind. Amen.

Attitude

Words can never adequately convey the incredible impact of our attitude toward life. The longer I live the more convinced I become that life is 10 percent what happens to us and 90 percent how we respond to it. . . .

I believe the single most significant decision I can make on a day-to-day basis is my choice of attitude. It is more important than my past, my education, my bankroll, my successes or failures, fame or pain, what other people think of me or say about me, my circumstances, or my position. Attitude is that "single string" that keeps me going or cripples my progress. It alone fuels my fire or assaults my hope. When my attitudes are right, there's no barrier too high, no valley too deep, no dream too

extreme, no challenge too great
for me.

—Chuck Swindoll in
Strengthening Your Grip (206–7)

We have cancer. The facts are undeniable. The real question is how we will respond to that news. Will we become bitter? Will we give up? Or will we determine to fight our disease, look for the positive, and live in hope?

Our attitude not only is a big factor in our healing but also helps give significance and meaning to our trials. Studies have shown that a positive attitude helps the healing process. But even more than that, it is the platform on which our hope, courage, and faith are exhibited. Attitude is our light set on a hill that speaks to a watching world of the reality of our Savior.

God of goodness, help me not to be ruled by circumstance but to learn to turn circumstance in my hand like a stone, looking for its most pleasing perspective. Give me the eyes to see the positive and the hopeful. Amen.

A Prayer in Time of Trouble

Don't punish me, LORD,
or even correct me
      when you are angry!
Have pity on me and heal
      my feeble body.
My bones tremble with fear,
and I am in deep distress.
      How long will it be?

Turn and come to my rescue.
Show your wonderful love
      and save me, LORD.
If I die, I cannot praise you
or even remember you.
My groaning has worn me out.
At night my bed and pillow
      are soaked with tears.

—Psalm 6:1-6, CEV

God our Helper, I need you.
I'm hurting and scared and lonely.
Please help me.
Give me the strength
to go through this ordeal. Amen.

The Hidden Time Bomb

Tick. Tick. Tick. My friend smiled at me and said, "I have a time bomb ticking away in me." His time bomb was prostate cancer, and his prognosis was not hopeful. Then he smiled again and said, "You do, too. None of us is immortal, you know." I was young and healthy and thought it an odd thing to say.

My friend was not trying to be morbid. He was trying to remind me of the truth that tomorrow is not guaranteed for any of us. Healthy though I seemed, I might leave his office and be hit by a car, struck by lightning, shot by a maniac, or catch Legionnaire's disease. All any of us know that we have is today. Some of us are much more painfully aware of that fact than are others.

Jesus was a today-oriented person. He taught, "Don't worry about tomorrow. It will take care of itself. You have enough to worry about today" (Matthew 6:34, CEV.) His point was not that since tomorrow is not guaranteed, we should live it up today. Rather, he was saying that today is the only day we have to live in faith and hope and kindness and love. Today is the only tableau on which we have to live our lives in the presence of God and to be a true human being.

This is true whether you have cancer now or not. Don't allow the weight of presumed or anticipated tomorrows steal today from you. As one cartoon character said, "I try to take one day at a time, but lately several days have been sneaking up on me together!"

Dear God, today I choose to have faith, to show love, to be courageous. I will not worry about tomorrow. Tomorrow is an unknown set of variables. When those variables are revealed, then I will have to face them with faith, love, and courage. That is the same opportunity that I am faced with now. Amen.

Pray

Don't worry about anything, but pray
about everything. With thankful hearts
offer up your prayers and requests to God.
—Philippians 4:6, CEV

Pray. Pray. Don't forget to pray. Prayer is no guarantee that you will get the answer you want. But con-
tinue to pray anyway.

Think about your children. In simple, childlike
faith they come to you with requests all the time.
Sometimes they ask for ice cream before supper,
and you have to say no. Sometimes they ask you
to make their goldfish come back to life, and you
are not able. But these nos do not stop them from
coming to you again the next day and asking for
something else. If the truth be told, even though
we do have to say no sometimes, we love to say yes.
We love to be able to give our children the desires
of their hearts. So does God.

I asked for healing of my cancer. God gave me healing—after a year of chemotherapy. Why the delay? I don't know. Children rarely do. Once, at a prayer meeting, I received a miraculous healing of the depression that I was in. I had been in that depression for a year. Why did God wait? I don't know that either. But the healing was supernatural.

Sometimes we forget to pray. The second time I had cancer, I started treatment with one oncologist, only to be severely dissatisfied. I found myself in the troubling position of being in the middle of a chemotherapy cycle, having a dangerous disease, and not having a clue about where to find a new oncologist. Somewhere I remembered to pray. Within a day or two God provided me with the most wonderful oncologist that I could have dreamed up for myself. God loves to say yes to his children.

Jesus, give me that simple, childlike faith
that believes and that continues to ask
even when sometimes the answer is no.
I do ask in the name of Jesus for my healing.
I also ask that you help me where I need help. Amen.

True Faith

There are a lot of people with mistaken notions about faith. Some people have the idea that we are not supposed to bother God with our problems. They think that if God wants to help, God will— whether we ask or not. They believe that God has already chosen whether to heal our cancer or not. On the opposite side are the ones who think that our faith is so vital and potent that if we don't get what we ask for, it is always our fault. They tell us, "If you would just believe hard enough, your cancer would be healed."

The best place to see what real faith is about is to look at Jesus. His prayer in the garden of Gethsemane shows us the correct balance. As Jesus faced the specter of the cross, his personal desire was to avoid the suffering. He didn't say, "Oh, God doesn't care about my personal desires." Rather, he took the desires of his heart to God. "Father, if you are willing, take this cup from me." He asked in faith for a miracle, believing wholeheartedly that God could deliver.

He asked . . . but he did not demand. He did not say, "I've asked; now you have to do it." Neither did he blame his own lack of faith when God said no. Perfect faith asks God, in trust that God can and will respond if it is for our best. But perfect faith leaves the final decision up to God. "Father, if you are willing, take this cup from me; yet not my will, but yours be done" (Luke 22:42, NIV).

*Lover of my soul, I bring the desires of my heart
to you in faith. Cancer is but a small thing
for you to heal. Help me to trust
whatever you have in mind for my life. Amen.*

God Can Be Trusted

Save me, God!
     I am about to drown.
I am sinking deep in the mud,
     and my feet are slipping.
I am about to be swept under
     by a mighty flood.
I am worn out from crying,
     and my throat is dry.
I have waited for you
     till my eyes are blurred.

But I pray to you, LORD.
     So when the time is right,
answer me and help me
     with your wonderful love.
Don't let me sink in the mud,
but save me from my enemies
     and from the deep water.

Don't let me be
  swept away by a flood
  or drowned in the ocean
  or swallowed by death.

— Psalm 69:1-3,13-15, CEV

Precious Lord, I have no one to help me but you.
You are a rock in the middle of a swirling flood.
I climb up on you and am safe. Amen.

Hero

Oftentimes people would call me a hero as they watched me go through my sufferings. I did not feel like a hero; I just desired to live. What we go through looks heroic to other people because they realize the depth of our trials and they are not sure they could hold up as well as we do. We appear to be managing with grace and strength and courage.

Of course, they do not see the times when we break down and cry. They do not see when we get into such a panic that we feel we might lose our minds. They do not see the depression and the pity parties we throw.

If other people want to call you a hero, let them. But don't hang around your neck the burden of trying to be a hero. Aim at surviving. If you survive with flair or courage, great. If you survive by the skin of your teeth, that's okay, too.

Some friends and I crossed a plank suspension footbridge over a gorge. Some of us crossed over skipping and laughing; others, nearly crawling and holding on with all their might. The important thing was that we all got across.

One of the most helpful cards I received when I was sick had a picture of Snoopy hanging from the edge of a cliff. The caption read, "Hang in there."

God my strength, in faith I will hang in there today.
I know that you are there to catch me if I fall.
My assurance comes not from my own
resources but from you. Amen.

An Invitation

I lived for a while in the mountains of east Tennessee, where almost all the houses had old, hand-dug wells. One summer we experienced a drought, and many people found themselves without water. The dry weather showed whose wells were adequately deep. Cancer does the same thing with our faith.

The first time I was diagnosed with cancer I thought I had a wonderful relationship with God and that I was jam-packed with faith. I was even a minister. But it didn't take long for me to be shown up for what I really was—a weak, scared, young man with a rather shallow relationship with God. When I cranked down the bucket for some comfort, I came up with dust.

Sometimes, to grow, we need to see our lack. I have come to see that experience as an invitation from God to dig deeper. If our faith is not deep enough to handle cancer, then it is not deep enough. My second bout with cancer ten years later was much less jarring because God had used my first experience to help me grow up. I had come to a firmer trust in the Lord. The water level was still a little low but not as shallow as before.

If your cancer has revealed to you that your faith was shallower than you thought, look at it as an invitation from God to drill down to a deeper reservoir.

Heavenly Father, I confess that I do not like to see my own weaknesses. I like to think that I am strong and capable. Help me to see my weaknesses not as failure but as an invitation to grow. Amen.

Loved Ones

As Jesus hung on the cross, he took care of an important piece of business—one that might have been neglected in the large work of saving the world. He took care of his family obligations. Looking down helplessly, he did what he could do and asked John, his disciple, to take care of his mother.

Often when we have cancer, we are not able to take care of our loved ones. We are too ill. When I had cancer, I helplessly watched my wife struggle to run a household by herself. I so much desired to mow the yard or fix the car but was unable. For a year I could not bounce my four-year-old on my lap. The main interaction I had with my eight-year-old was to ask him to bring me the throw-up bucket.

It is immensely painful to have to stand by your loved ones and watch as they flounder. We need to be able to do what Jesus did: transfer responsibility. This might be to friends or family, as Jesus did. Friends from our church took over mowing the yard and fixing the car. Grandparents gave extra love and care to the kids.

We can also transfer responsibility to God. Sometimes we act like practical atheists, thinking that if we don't do it, it won't get done. We can pray in faith and ask God to watch over our children and rear them with the Spirit's protection. Ask God to keep this traumatic event from crippling them. Ask God to uphold our spouse and be his or her substitute helpmate—for supernatural strength to be poured forth.

It does no good to beat up ourselves for something we are helpless to do. Even Jesus knew his limitations and needed others' help.

God my help, I turn to you. I have never been as strong or as in control as I imagined. You have been there watching and protecting my family all along. Give me faith to see that truth. Amen.

A Prayer for the Lord's Help

How much longer, LORD,
    will you forget about me?
Will it be forever?
    How long will you hide?
How long must I be confused
    and miserable all day?
How long will my enemies
    keep beating me down?

Please listen, LORD God,
    and answer my prayers.
Make my eyes sparkle again,
or else I will fall
    into the sleep of death.
My enemies will say,
    "Now we've won!"
They will be greatly pleased
    when I am defeated.

I trust your love,
and I feel like celebrating
        because you rescued me.
You have been good to me, LORD,
        and I will sing about you.

—Psalm 13, CEV

God, it feels as if you have forgotten me.
That is the worst feeling in the world.
I fight my feelings. I choose to trust in the sun
even when all I see are clouds. Amen.

Why, God?

A few years ago I witnessed a scene that helped me to picture how our suffering looks from God's perspective. I was visiting a young couple whose four-month-old baby, Stephen, was in the hospital with liver failure. It's a hard thing to see young parents standing around a crib in a hospital, wearing gowns and masks, stroking their baby.

What happened next was horrifying. A nurse came in to draw blood. She asked the father to hold Stephen while she did her procedure. As I watched, Dad, tight-lipped, held the baby, knowing that drawing blood would hurt Stephen. As the needle went in, Stephen screamed out in pain. He looked up into his daddy's eyes and wailed in a way that could only mean, "Why are you doing this to me? Please stop!"

Helplessly, the father looked back into his eyes, trying to comfort Stephen, knowing that there was no way that he could explain that this was for the baby's good, fighting back his own tears of love and

sympathy, and hoping that Stephen trusted enough
in his love to believe in him. That is the same way
that God looks at us as we cry out, uncomprehend-
ing, in our pain.

Father in heaven, it is a confession of faith
that I look into your eyes and trust, despite my pain,
that you love me and are doing all you can for me.
Keep me looking into your eyes. Amen.

Miracles

You're in a terrible way, at the end of your rope, in an impossible situation? This may sound a bit crazy at first . . . but that qualifies you as material for a miracle. When we read the Bible we find that the first requirement for a miracle to occur is that people have run out of human options. They absolutely know that they need God. Without God, whatever they need will not occur.

A crowd of at least five thousand people has gathered in a remote place to hear Jesus teach. They have stayed past mealtime, until they are so hungry that some of them will faint before they reach a town. The disciples are concerned. "Send the people away," they urge. Jesus says, "You feed them." "Impossible," reply the disciples. Jesus smiles. He knows that the situation is now ripe for a miracle.

The people of Israel are fleeing the armies of Pharaoh. They come to the edge of the Red Sea and stop. Why has Moses led them here? They look behind and see the Egyptians. Trapped, they are panic-stricken. God smiles. Now they are ready for a miracle.

Is your situation hopeless? Now is your opportunity to ask God for a miracle. Ask for his help. Tell God that when he acts, you won't attribute your cure to anyone else—you will give all the glory to God. Stand still, and see the salvation of the Lord.

Lord of hosts, I stand helpless before your throne,
a humble supplicant. There is no one else to turn to.
Only you can help. I wait for you to move
your right hand of power. Amen.

Answered Prayer

I asked God for strength,
        that I might achieve,
    I was made weak,
            that I might learn humbly to obey . . .
I asked for health,
        that I might do greater things,
    I was given infirmity,
            that I might do better things . . .
I asked for riches,
        that I might be happy,
    I was given poverty,
            that I might be wise. . .
I asked for power,
        that I might have the praise of men,
    I was given weakness,
            that I might feel the need of God . . .
I asked for all things,
        that I might enjoy life,
    I was given life,
            that I might enjoy all things . . .

I got nothing that I asked for —
but everything I had hoped for;
> Almost despite myself,
> my unspoken prayers were answered.
>> I am among all men most richly blessed.

—Unknown Confederate soldier

O God, let me receive from you
that which you give.
Allow me to trust in your gifts.
Give me eyes to see them. Amen.

A Prayer for Help

Only you, LORD,
     are a mighty rock!
Don't refuse to help me
     when I pray.
If you don't answer me,
     I will soon be dead.
Please listen to my prayer
     and my cry for help,
as I lift my hands
     toward your holy temple.

You give strength
     to your people, LORD,
and you save and protect
     your chosen ones.
Come save us and bless us.
Be our shepherd and always
     carry us in your arms.

—Psalm 28:1-2,8-9, CEV

O Lord, I am glad that there is an ear
to listen when I cry out to heaven.
The One who formed the universe
is sympathetic to my plight.
I wait on your help, Father,
like a little child. Amen.

Joy

> You and I were created for joy, and
> if we miss it, we miss the reason for our
> existence. . . . If our joy is honest joy, it
> must somehow be congruous with
> human tragedy. This is the test of
> joy's integrity: is it compatible with
> pain? . . . Only the heart that hurts
> has a right to joy.
> —Lewis Smedes in *How Can It Be
> All Right When Everything Is All
> Wrong?*

Someone said that happiness is linked to happen-
ings. It is circumstance-based. If I feel good, I am
happy. If it's a nice, sunny day, I am happy. If
things are going my way, I am happy. Happiness
is not bad. In heaven we will be eternally happy
because our circumstances will be eternally pleas-
ant. Here on earth, however, is a different story.

Our circumstances can easily change, and our happiness runs out. Cancer comes, and it is often impossible to feel happy.

That's why the Bible doesn't talk much about happiness. Rather, it talks about joy. Joy is not circumstance-based; it is relationship-based. Joy is a gift from God. First Thessalonians 1:6 says, "In spite of severe suffering, you welcomed the message with the joy given by the Holy Spirit" (NIV). Joy was given. Joy came in spite of severe suffering. And joy was received. Joy is an attitude, as opposed to an emotion, that God gives us. It is an attitude of gratitude—not for the circumstance but for God who is with us in every circumstance. Paul Sailhamer has said, "Joy is that deep settled confidence that God is in control of every area of my life."

Stop grasping for happiness. Start receiving joy. Why? Because God with all his power and love is upholding you this second.

O Lord, I look past the circumstance into your face. I see love etched there. Because of that, I will rejoice. Amen.

No Help

A great aloneness settled upon me. I was on the phone with someone I trusted and respected, someone I turned to in times of trouble. He had often been of great help. When cancer and chemotherapy and chaos descended, I scrambled for help, calling friends and relatives. Little help was to be found, so in desperation I called Jap. He was kind; he was sympathetic; he gave all that he had to give.

But somewhere in the middle of the conversation it hit me. Cancer is something that no one can magically remove from you. Chemotherapy is something no one else can take for you. And death is something that no one else can face for you. The blackness of despair settled on me: "I'm all alone."

I interrupted Jap's consoling words, "Sorry to bother you, Jap. I guess that there's nothing you can really do, is there?" Jap was honest, "No, there's not." Then he added, "But it's still good to have friends. You don't need to go through this alone."

I was right, and he was right. No one can take away our personal trials. There are some things we have to face for ourselves. But it's still good to have friends, to at least have someone walk to the edge of our personal pit with us and be waiting for us when we return. Friends might not be saviors, but take all of them that you can get.

Heavenly Friend, there are things that only you can help me with. There are places that only you can show me through. Thank you for being there. And thank you for the earthly friends who can walk with me to the edge. Amen.

Faith

Sweeping across Germany at the end of
World War II, Allied forces searched
farms and houses looking for snipers. At
one abandoned house, almost a heap of
rubble, searchers with flashlights found
their way to the basement. There, on the
crumbling wall, a victim of the
Holocaust had scratched a star of David.
And beneath it, in rough lettering, the
message:

I believe in the Sun—
        even when it does not shine;
I believe in love—
        even when it is not shown;
I believe in God—
        even when he does not speak.

                    —Robert Schuller,
                "The Hour of Power."

We believe in the sun even when it does not shine because sometime, somewhere we have seen it before. We have seen that it exists and that our lack of perception of it does not make it cease to exist. On the overcast days we rely on our experience to affirm the sun's reality. We know that if we could board a plane and fly up through the clouds, there the sun would be in all its glory.

Sometimes we must do the same with God. There are times—especially when we suffer—when we cannot see or feel God. In these times we must rely on the memory of those times when we were very much aware of the presence of God in our lives. Suffering can act as a dense cloud to block out our perception of God. Like this Holocaust victim, we must exercise memory and faith to see God shining like the sun behind the clouds.

I believe; help my unbelief, O Lord.
Help me to flex my muscles of faith,
to join the long line of those who have
believed without seeing. Amen.

Suffering and Praise

My God, my God, why have you
          deserted me?
Why are you so far away?
Won't you listen to my groans
          and come to my rescue?
I cry out day and night,
but you don't answer,
          and I can never rest.

Yet you are the holy God,
ruling from your throne
          and praised by Israel.
Our ancestors trusted you,
          and you rescued them.
When they cried out for help,
          you saved them,
and you did not let them down
          when they depended on you.

—Psalm 22:1-5, CEV

Master, you feel far away.
I know that my feelings
don't dictate where you are.
My feelings don't change the truth
that you are near and that you care
with an everlasting care. Amen.

Prejudice

God is prejudiced. Prejudice means to prejudge based on a trait—to lump together all people with a certain characteristic. The Bible tells us that God is favorably prejudiced toward all who are weak, downtrodden, and hurting. Read of this divine prejudice:

> For the Lord . . . will have compassion on his afflicted ones. (Isaiah 49:13, NIV)

> He does not ignore the cry of the afflicted. (Psalm 9:12, NIV)

> But God, who comforts the downcast, comforted us . . .
> (2 Corinthians 7:6, NIV)

> You hear, O LORD, the desire of the afflicted; you encourage them, and you listen to their cry. (Psalm 10:17, NIV)

> "For the Son of Man came to seek and to save what was lost."
> (Luke 19:10, NIV)

> He will take pity on the weak and the
> needy and save the needy from death.
> He will rescue them from oppression
> and violence, for precious is their blood
> in his sight.
>
> (Psalm 72:13-14, NIV)

> "Come to me, all you who are weary
> and burdened, and I will give you rest."
> (Matthew 11:28, NIV)

Do you see that God does not differentiate? The
Lord says, Come, all who are weary. God is a God
who comforts the downcast. No other characteristics are named. Are you needy and hurting? Know
that God is biased toward you.

*Being needy, God, I know that I am a special recipient
of your care. Thank you for your love that flows
by the depth of my need for it. I praise you. Amen.*

Where Is God?

Does it feel as if God is not with you? Not in the neighborhood? Maybe even left the country? That is a common feeling when you're suffering. I remember strongly feeling that way once when I was in the hospital. I was so overwhelmed with a feeling of cosmic loneliness that I went to see the chaplain. "I'm a Christian," I explained to him, "but it feels like God is a million miles away."

He directed me to the book of Job and asked me if I thought that Job ever felt that way. The book of Job is about a man who went through extreme suffering—not because he was evil and not because God sent suffering upon him but because he was a good and righteous man and Satan wanted to torment him. God seems to have decided to use Satan's torment to bring his beloved Job to a deeper faith and dependence on God.

But Job didn't know any of that. He only knew that he was miserable. And, yes, he felt that God was a million miles away. He cried out, "If only I knew where to find him" (Job 23:3, NIV). The chaplain then asked me another question: "At what point did God leave Job?"

Leave him? I realized then that, despite all of Job's feelings of desertion, God had never left him. If anything, God was closer to Job in his suffering than at any other time.

Heavenly Father, I so much wish that I could make you materialize in front of me and sweep away all my doubts.
But I know that your Word talks about faith.
I know that this is the time to exercise my faith and trust that you are there. Amen.

The Unreliability of Feelings

Have you ever felt that God has disappeared, doesn't care, has turned against you? Job felt many of those feelings. He said, "I long for the past, when God took care of me" (Job 29:1, CEV). And he cried out, "God has turned brutal, stirring up a windstorm to toss me about" (Job 30:21-22, CEV). Job felt that God was no longer his friend, that God had changed in his relationship to Job, that God had even turned brutal. Looking from afar, we can see that that was not the case. We know that God was hovering by, watching his servant tenderly.

But it is also true that when we're Job, when pain and suffering are our daily bread, it is easy to feel those same things. The truth is that those are real feelings. But feelings can be both real and unreliable at the same time.

When airplanes were first invented, there was very little instrumentation. Pilots flew by sight and sensation. When they would gain or lose altitude, they would feel more or less pressure as their body pressed against or lifted off the seat. This was called "flying by the seat of your pants," flying by feeling rather than by scientific gauges. The problem was that often the pilots' sensations were not accurate. Many pilots crashed because of the unreliability of their feelings. Learn to acknowledge your feelings but to distrust them when they go against God's Word.

You are true, O God. My feelings do not make you disappear. Your existence does not depend upon my sensations. Give me faith to trust in you more than in my feelings. Amen.

Skin and Bones

I am skin and bones—
      just barely alive.
My friends, I beg you for pity!
      God has made me his target.
Hasn't he already done enough?
      Why do you join the attack?

I wish that my words
could be written down
      or chiseled into rock.
I know that my Savior lives,
and at the end
      he will stand on this earth.
My flesh may be destroyed,
yet from this body
      I will see God.
Yes, I will see him for myself,
      and I long for that moment.

—Job 19:20-27, CEV

O God, I am so confused.
My mind can't think straight.
One moment I think you are against me;
the next I remember that you are my Redeemer.
Help me to hold onto that thought—
that one day I shall see you
for who you really are. Amen.

Mystery

The tendency of the cancer to recur was
held at bay or perhaps even wiped out
by my will to live, by a new love, by
new interests, by immunotherapy, maybe
by hepatitis, maybe by good fortune,
maybe by God. . . . I give respectable
scientific methods the credit due and
reserve for the unknown factors the
awesome name of mystery which I
refuse to confuse with science.
    —Morris Abram in *The Day Is Short:
        An Autobiography* (222–23)

There is so much mystery when it comes to the
human body. Mysteries about how much the mind
can affect the body. Mysteries about the origin of
cancer. Mysteries about environmental effects.
Mysteries about the spiritual world. Don't think
that the treatment of your disease is all a cut-and-

dried science. There is science to it. But an honest physician will tell you that there are many unknown variables. Every doctor has had to concede to those variables at some point. Someone who should have survived doesn't. Someone who was pronounced a goner lives to rock his or her great-grandchildren. Besides all to-be-discovered earthly variables, there is God.

Fight the disease with medicine and with hope. Supplement your medical treatment with alternative treatments. Try an exercise program or envisioning health. Maybe you will stumble on one of those mysterious cures. And maybe that cure will even come in the hope that comes from trying something that in itself is not helpful. Most of all remember prayer. Science has not yet fathomed the power of God.

God of the universe, forgive me when I inadvertently act like an atheist. You have made this world much more complex than we humans have yet discovered. And you yourself are able at any moment to completely confound our limited analysis. Amen.

Listening to Your Body

"Your body will talk to you. Listen to it." Those were the words of a friend who was battling prostate cancer. At first I thought them peculiar. But the longer I lived with cancer, the stronger I heard the voice of my body. "You are overexerting me. Please rest a while." "Yes, you may take me to the office today, but work only at two-thirds speed." "I need some exercise. I need to feel alive!" "I can take a lot of chemotherapy punishment, but there are lines of no return."

You do well to listen to the voice of your body. As much as you are able, give it what it needs. Our bodies will subliminally lead us to what we need. We will begin to crave certain foods, sunlight, rest, company. Sometimes our bodies will even help us in medication choices.

I remember a time when I was in a deep depression. I was undergoing some harsh chemotherapy.

In an attempt to help, my oncologist was prescribing several antidepressants and tranquilizers, but I sank deeper and deeper into despair. One day, my oncologist's partner was on call and came to visit me at the hospital. When she looked over my chart and talked to me, she observed that the medicines might be making me too drugged and lethargic, that maybe less medicine and more physical exercise would help.

I was caught between differing opinions of two excellent physicians. Who really knew which would be better? But my body knew. When she spoke of fewer pills and more exercise, my body nearly shouted yes. I immediately put her alternate plan into action and did much better emotionally.

Heavenly Father, I am fearfully and wonderfully made. You yourself knit me together. Help me to listen to and hear the voice of my body. Amen.

Pressure

Someone said, "When pressure comes, it can either push you away from Jesus or press you into his bosom." It is our choice what we allow trials to do to us. Suffering can make you bitter or better—it depends on whether you reach out to God or allow bitterness to take root. Job's wife asked, "Why do you still trust God? Why don't you curse him and die?" But Job replied, "Don't talk like a fool! If we accept blessings from God, we must accept trouble as well" (Job 2:9-10, CEV).

Outside of God there is bitterness, utter aloneness, despair, death. We can choose to let the pressure push us there. But it is a choice. We can also choose to let it push us close to God, helpless and hurting, looking for the grace that is sufficient even in our weakest hour.

When King David got into rough situations, he knew where to turn. He allowed the trial to act as a G-force that pressed him hard unto God and held him there through all the spins, turns, and loop-de-loops of life.

Heavenly Friend, let this trial strengthen
our relationship. Let it make me so dependent on you
that you are my all and everything. Let me be
so squeezed to you that we are inseparable. Amen.

Prayer of Desperation

About this time, Hezekiah got sick and was almost dead. Isaiah the prophet went in and told him, "The LORD says you won't ever get well. You are going to die, so you had better start doing what needs to be done."

Hezekiah turned toward the wall and prayed, "Don't forget that I have been faithful to you, LORD. I have obeyed you with all of my heart, and I do whatever you say is right." After this, he cried hard.

Before Isaiah got to the middle court of the palace, the LORD sent him back to Hezekiah with this message:

> Hezekiah, you are the ruler of my
> people, and I am the LORD God, who
> was worshiped by your ancestor David.
> I heard you pray, and I saw you cry. I
> will heal you, so that three days from
> now you will be able to worship in my

temple. I will let you live fifteen years more, while I protect you and your city from the king of Assyria. . . .

Then Isaiah said to the king's servants, "Bring some mashed figs and place them on the king's open sore. He will then get well."

—2 Kings 20:1-7, CEV

O God, like Hezekiah, I cry out to you. Hear my prayers and see my tears and heal me. You are the God who listens to the cries of your people. Amen.

Friends

Friends—we all need them. How beautiful they are when they come to us in times of need. A meal dropped by, a phone call, a visit, a little kindness. And cards from near and far. "Just thinking of you." "Hope you get well." "You're special to us."

It's overwhelming to think about. People think of us, hurt for us, want to help us. They take time from their busy schedules to drive to the drugstore. They linger over the cards looking for the right one to say what their hearts feel. Put out hard-earned cash. Write a little something extra. The time, the thought, the care. How they uplift us. "More than kisses, letters mingle souls," wrote John Donne.

And sometimes, absolute strangers—people who care for us without ever having met us. "We heard from a mutual acquaintance that you weren't doing well, and we just had to sit down and write you a note." Amazing. Kindness almost divine. To reach across the chasm of strangerhood and send love, sympathy, a word in season. Old friends and new friends—God bless them all.

God, you created us to be in community.
You said, "It is not good for the man to be alone."
Thank you for the friends you have brought my way.
I will cherish them. Amen.

Emotionally Handicapped Friends

Some people are not emotionally strong enough to deal with your illness. They will give quick, pat answers. They will change the subject. They will avoid you. They will come so emotionally unglued that you end up having to care for them. Some relatives who called me would get so upset about my situation that I had to spend the whole phone call comforting and reassuring them even though I desperately needed someone to comfort and reassure me.

Forgive them for their lack. You are needy, and it hurts to not have that need met. But it does no good wishing for a world that is not. Recognize that it is not that they don't care. It is rather that they do not know how to care or that they are so afraid of disease or anything related to dying that they are unable to care.

My father was so poor in knowing how to deal with his own feelings that whenever we would speak on the phone he would stick to a safe subject such as fishing or sports. When he wouldn't ask how I was doing, it hurt my feelings. But other relatives told me that he would hang up and sob. When I finally confronted him, he told me that he was afraid that it would upset me for him to cry. I explained to him that sometimes I needed for him to cry with me. He began to learn how to help. But it didn't come naturally.

Not everybody can handle emotions in a way that is helpful to you. Know that. Forgive that. Learn to overlook that. And seek out the people who are strong, someone you can lean on emotionally.

Loving Lord, thank you that I can turn to you
even when there is no one else to turn to.
Help me to not expect people to be you.
Help me to forgive them for their weaknesses,
just as I need forgiveness for mine. Amen.

You Collected My Tears

> You have seen me tossing and turning
> through the night. You have collected
> all my tears and preserved them in your
> bottle! You have recorded every one in
> your book.
>
> —Psalm 56:8, TLB

Many are the tears of the cancer patient. Tears on hearing a positive diagnosis. Tears at the cold statistics: "You have a 50/50 chance." Tears at the thought of leaving loved ones. Tears at the losses even if you survive—a breast, fertility, eyesight. Tears for all the emotional trauma and physical pain.

Even Jesus cried. When his friend Lazarus died, he felt the weight of the sorrow of his friends. Sometimes the sadness of life is best expressed by tears.

The promise of God is that our tears are precious to him. He cries with us when we cry. Our tears are not lost. They are collected and preserved, every one, in God's bottle. They are recorded in his book. Some day, when we go to heaven, we will see in the household of God a bottle with our name on it—a vial of remembrance for God and a memorial of his love for us and the pain that he shared with us.

I give my tears to you, O God. They are the cries
of one who is in a broken and hurting land.
You have walked in our shoes and know full well
our sorrows. You comfort us. Amen.

Jesus Knows

We are people of flesh and blood.
That is why Jesus became
      one of us.
He died to destroy the devil,
      who had power over death.
But he also died to rescue
      all of us who live each day
      in fear of dying.

He had to be one of us,
so that he could serve God
      as our merciful and faithful high priest
and sacrifice himself
      for the forgiveness of our sins.
And now that Jesus has suffered and was
tempted,
he can help anyone else
      who is tempted.

—Hebrews 2:14-15,17-18, CEV

Heavenly Friend, I am so glad that you know
what it is like to walk in my shoes.
You suffered as I am,
and your flesh experienced the emotions
that swirl through my soul.
So you know how much I need
your divine help. Amen.

Pain Is Temporary

Pain is temporary. When I was four years old, I knocked over an iron, spilling out the steaming water on my arm. It was painful. I cried. It is my first memory of life. But the memory has changed. At first it was a dreadful memory—one that is the stuff of nightmares. Then it took on a dullness that comes with time. Now it is an amusing anecdote.

Your present sufferings are such. Though they don't feel like it now, eventually their power to cause you pain by the memory of them will fade. There will come a day when you will look back and laugh. Each time I had cancer it has taken time—two or three years—but the memories eventually lost their power. Speak to your pain out loud and say, "You are only temporary. Someday you will pass."

Lord, I will speak to my pain.
I will speak life. Pain consumes me
so that it feels as if it is all there is.
But I choose to look beyond
to better days with you. Amen.

Pain as a Pointer

Pain is everywhere, even in wellness. We voluntarily put ourselves through many kinds of pain and discomfort. The grunt of overindulgence at the Thanksgiving dinner. "I wish I hadn't eaten that last piece of pie a la mode." The boyish pleasure in getting sore from too much exercise or the bruises from playing football with the guys in the park. Frying ourselves in cooking oil at the beach to have a nice tan. Driving all night long to get to a favorite vacation destination. Drinking ourselves sick or to a hangover. Dieting. Eating spicy foods on top of an ulcer. All the various work pains from hunching over a word processor to running a jack hammer to spending the day in high heels.

Pain is a part of life. It is earth this side of paradise. Oh, there are many pleasures too, but even in our pleasures we have trouble avoiding some degree of pain. Even pain can speak to us of the lack of total satisfaction to be found here on earth. It turns our souls toward the one who has "gone to prepare for us a better place."

Lord, thank you even for the pain. It reminds me
that I am not at my final place of destination.
I am just a pilgrim on my way
to somewhere much better. Amen.

No More Suffering

Pain is temporary. If nothing else it will end when this life ends. For the believer pain is not a part of the next phase of existence. "There will be no more death or mourning or crying or pain, for the old order of things has passed away" (Revelation 21:4, NIV). Not only can we not take our toys or our money with us when we go, but also we will not be able to take our pain. It will be extra baggage that we leave along the trail to the light of God.

This is our hope when all other hope is gone. It is not a hope that makes us give up on this world. But it is a hope, like the ace up one's sleeve, that we can pull out when the hand we're holding is not a winner. Sometimes there is nothing else in this world to hope for—just a maddening continuation of the downward spiral. It's then that we hold on, not to be well again in this world, but for a better world. The apostle Paul wrote, "I consider that our present sufferings are not worth comparing with the glory that will be revealed in us" (Romans 8:18, NIV).

We are no longer in Eden and not yet in paradise. Even if by some miracle we would be healed, we would be healed only to die again. Jesus said that in this life there will be tribulation. Thank God that he has promised to take us to where he is.

Father, forgive me when I forget that
my true home is not here and now.
Like Jesus, I despise the pain,
but I endure it for the glory set before me.
Help me to cling to the true hope
of the Christian. Amen.

The Good Shepherd

You, LORD, are my shepherd.
> I will never be in need.
You let me rest in fields
> of green grass.
You lead me to streams
of peaceful water,
> and you refresh my life.

You are true to your name,
and you lead me
> along the right paths.
I may walk through valleys
as dark as death,
> but I won't be afraid.
You are with me,
and your shepherd's rod
> makes me feel safe.

—Psalm 23:1-4, CEV

Comfort me, O God.
Hold me to your chest
as a shepherd cuddles a lamb.
Let me fall asleep
in your arms. Amen.

Bloom Where You Are Planted

Don't like where life has put you right now? The book of Acts tells us that one day Paul and Silas were mauled in a riot, stripped and beaten by the police, and then thrown into jail. As dark came on, they could have thrown a giant pity party. They could have sat in despair, saying, "This stinks!"

Instead they believed that they were where they were by divine appointment. They chose to bloom where they were planted, no matter how infertile the soil looked. They sang hymns and praised God. They must have been a witness to their fellow prisoners and certainly to their jailer, whom they later led to Christ.

Can you choose to believe the same about where you are? That even though Satan has brought you there for ill, God has brought you there to bear light? You may be hooked up to IVs receiving your chemotherapy, and there is someone in the chair next to you. You may be in the hospital, and the nurses are your mission field. Or your coworkers may be looking on as you struggle to do your work.

It may not come naturally, but ask God to help you to live a life of praise and thanksgiving, wearing a good attitude, and to bloom where you are planted.

O God, I have not moved out of your domain.
I confess that your sovereign hand has brought me
to where I am for some purpose.
Fill me with your Spirit that I might
bear your reflection. Amen.

The Refiner's Fire

He sat by a furnace of sevenfold heat
    As he watched by the precious ore,
And closer he bent with a searching gaze
    As he heated it more and more.

He knew he had ore that could stand the test
    And he wanted the finest gold,
To mold as a crown for the King to wear,
    Set with gems of price untold.

So he laid our gold in the burning fire,
    Tho' we fain would say him, "Nay";
And watched the dross that we had not seen,
    As it melted and passed away.

And the gold grew brighter and yet more bright,
    But our eyes were dim with tears,
We saw but the fire—not the Master's hand,
    And questioned with anxious fears.

Yet our gold shone out with a richer glow
    As it mirrored a Form above,
That bent o're the fire, tho' unseen by us,
    With a look of ineffable love.

Can we think it pleases his loving heart
  to cause us a moment's pain?
Ah, no, but he sees through the present cross
  The bliss of eternal gain.

    So he waited there with watchful eye
      With a love that is strong and sure,
    And his gold did not suffer a bit more heat
      Than was needed to make it pure.

        —Author unknown

Then I will purify them
  and put them to the test,
just as gold and silver
  are purified and tested.

      — Zechariah 13:9, CEV

O God, I feel the heat of your transforming process.
Sometimes it feels as if I will burn up and
wither away. But your hand and your eye are
steady and sure. Do your work in my soul. Amen.

Bottled Anger

Do you ever feel angry with God? Job did. He said, "I am desperate because God All-Powerful refuses to do what is right" (Job 27:2, CEV). What should we do when we feel angry with God, when we feel that God has done us dirty or that God needs our forgiveness for the rotten way he has treated us? Should we bottle up those feelings, pretend that they're not there, and put on a false face of "praise the Lord"? Some people do. They don't want to sin by telling God what they really feel.

Job did two remarkable things with those feelings. First, he was comfortable enough in his relationship with God that he felt he could express his real emotions. They weren't pretty emotions. But he felt that God could handle the truth. Isn't how much honesty we feel free to express a gauge of the depth of our relationship with a person?

The second remarkable thing is that God did not reject Job for his angry outburst. God did not cast down a lightning bolt. God did sit down and have a serious talk with Job. God did tell Job that there was a lot about the universe that he couldn't begin to explain to Job. But God did not appear to be terribly irritated with Job. As a matter of fact, God was much more angry with Job's friends who counseled him to deny and bottle up his feelings.

My God, I confess that I am a mess.
I have all sorts of unreasonable emotions
that I don't know what to do with.
I even have anger toward you.
Lord, I lift this tangled mess up to you.
Please help me to sort it out. Amen.

Can't Find God

I cannot find God anywhere—
in front or back of me,
        to my left or my right.
God is always at work,
        though I never see him.
But he knows what I am doing,
and when he tests me,
        I will be as pure as gold.
I have never refused to follow
        any of his commands,
and I have always treasured
        his teachings.
But he alone is God,
        and who can oppose him?
God does as he pleases,
and he will do exactly
        what he intends with me.

Merely the thought
of God All-Powerful
        makes me tremble with fear.

—Job 23:8-16, CEV

I wish I could break through the haze
and find you, God. In my heart of hearts
I know that you are there, but it feels
as if you have gone on vacation.
Help me to muddle through the darkness. Amen.

Honesty

[We need] to honestly tell God how we feel. He can handle our authentic cries of pain and disappointment. He can even help us work through them. . . .

What I've learned is that often these authentic outpourings of frustration, or even anger, are necessary steps on the path to wholeness. The cathartic process of pouring our hearts out to the Lord, of emptying ourselves of pent-up emotions and unanswered questions, opens the way for insight and understanding.

The same thing happens to us that so often happened to the psalmist. After the outburst comes the renewed perspective. The lights go on. We realize anew that in spite of the heartache or the unanswered questions, God is still God. There is still hope. We still matter to Him. The Holy Spirit still lives in us. The Bible is still true. The church is still intact. Heaven still awaits. And in that we can rejoice.

—From *Honest to God* by Bill Hybels

O Master, part of our humanness
is to have emotions that are not easily tamed.
They spring out suddenly
from unseen sources
like whales rising from the deep.
Thank you for loving us in our frailty. Amen.

Darkness

When we read the story of Joseph in the Bible, we see a steady spiral downward. Perhaps you're feeling that spiral in your life. Joseph starts as a precocious son. Gets sold as a slave. Gets falsely accused of rape. And ends up in a deep, dark dungeon. It must have felt like a freefall into the blackness.

But as we read the story, we see a man who did not let his circumstances dictate his inner attitude. At each downward spiral he chose to live in faith and hope. Joseph was in the darkness, but he did not allow the darkness to get into him. Joseph was in prison, but he didn't allow himself to be a prisoner of cynicism or bitterness or despair.

It is easy to let where you are be in control of who you are. Faith is the choice to live ignoring the outer stimuli, to see God. And seeing God, to know that there is hope. Cancer has driven you into a prison of illness, hospital rooms, doctors' clinics, a sickbed. That is where you are. It can be a dark place. But choose not to let the darkness get into you. Choose not to be a prisoner. Your spirit always has the option to be free.

O God, like a nightmare the darkness chases me.
I can feel it just over my shoulder, waiting for me
to give in to its gloom. I choose to live in your light.
Dispel the darkness like the rising sun. Amen.

Time

The unbearable weight and monotony of time. The slow ticking of the clock in the hospital room, especially on the days when there are no visitors. The incredibly long afternoons of vegetating, too sick to work, read, take a walk, or even watch TV. The sleepless nights when the world is asleep except for you and the early-edition news anchors and the hawkers on the home shopping network.

The psalmist cries out, "How long, O God, how long?" How long, indeed. Time can feel like an enemy. Waiting can rob us of all morale. It's not just trouble and turmoil that deplete us. It's the passage of time without letup. Wouldn't it be great if we got to take vacations from our illness?

The Bible talks about two kinds of time. *Chronos* is the normal ticking of the clock that we have been describing. *Kairos* is a time of great import, pregnant with possibility, a time of culmination. The Bible sets great store in waiting patiently, hopefully, and expectantly through the hours, days, and years of *chronos* time until God in his mercy grants the *kairos* hour: Moses forty years in the wilderness; Joseph seven years in prison; Anna a lifetime of waiting for the consolation of Israel; Noah one hundred years building the ark. Seek to find the faithful serendipity of waiting.

Creator, Sustainer, Healer, give me the patience to bear the weight of time. Faithfulness has to do with all those empty hours until I see you act. Teach me what it means to wait on you. Amen.

The Past

I long for the past,
      when God took care of me,
and the light from his lamp
showed me the way
      through the dark.
I was in the prime of life,
God All-Powerful
      was my closest friend,
and all my children
      were nearby.

I felt certain that I would live
a long and happy life,
      then die in my own bed.
In those days I was strong
      like a tree with deep roots
and with plenty of water,
      or like an archer's new bow.

—Job 29:1-5,18-20, CEV

O Lord, help me to fight these black feelings.
I cannot seem to control
the dark thoughts that cloud my mind.
Hold me even in my times
of deep depression. Amen.

Chemotherapy Day

Chemotherapy day. The day that I've been dreading since I recovered from the last chemotherapy day. Even the thought of having the IVs hooked up makes me nauseous. Every bit of remaining sanity is screaming, "Run, run, run, and don't look back." Some do run. Is it courage that they do? Is it courage that I don't? For me, it's not courage but the desire to avoid the alternative. I try to enjoy my last hours of relative wellness, but a sense of foreboding hangs over me.

There is something ahead to be endured—as Jesus endured the cross. He didn't like or love the thought of going to the cross. The book of Hebrews says that for the joy set before him he endured the cross, despising the shame (Hebrews 12:2). The joy set before me is hopeful healing. So I will endure the nausea and the side effects.

And because the drugs are necessary to my recovery, I will do my best to envision them in a good light—an invading army of crusaders come to conquer the cancer cells, come to recapture the holy temple of my body. Today is chemotherapy day. That means one day, one battle closer to my liberation. I don't go to the battle with joy, but I am thankful that there is a battle to fight.

God, help me to find that for which I can be thankful.
Help me to keep positive — to see the harshness
of the drugs as a death knell to the cancer cells.
I thank you that I am one step closer to healing. Amen.

Courage

Courage is to live,
to not die before we die,
to open our eyes in the morning
and choose to keep them open,

to allow our mind to think —
even though those first morning thoughts
have the feel of a nightmare
not quite over —

to put pills down our throats
that we madly wish
to throw out the window,
removing the side effects,

to do today that which we are able
and to go through this day even
if being alive is the sum
of what we accomplish.

God, our provider,
provide me with the courage
that I need today. Heroes come in many forms.
The rest of us see only the end product.
It is a result of getting out of bed
on a day like today. Amen.

Sacrifice of Praise

> Through Jesus, therefore, let us continu-
> ally offer to God a sacrifice of praise—
> the fruit of lips that confess his name.
> —Hebrews 13:15, NIV

What is a sacrifice? In the Bible God always asked that something precious be sacrificed. Usually it was a living thing, the best and most perfect, such as a lamb without blemish. When you sacrificed it, there must have always been to some extent the thought, "I wouldn't mind keeping this. I could get some good use out of this. It is a personal loss to give this up."

The writer of Hebrews talks about a "sacrifice of praise." Sometimes praise is a rather easy sacrifice. All is good. We are blessed. The storehouse is full. Then it is only a little bit of ego we sacrifice when we say it is all from God.

I heard Joni Eareckson Tada, who suffered a diving accident at age seventeen that left her a quadriplegic for life, talk about the other times when praise does not come easily. When there is nothing inside of us that feels like praising. When all the outward circumstances dictate against praising. Joni said that these are the times when praise costs us something. We must work at praise. We must conquer all doubts and fears and say through gritted teeth, "I will praise God because God is worthy of praise."

Then she asked, "Which praise do you think blesses the heart of God more?" Sometimes I have praised God with so little emotion, all the while fighting every impulse of my human nature that I have felt guilty for my measly offering. But isn't that a tremendously beautiful offering as seen from the Father above?

God of glory, I do praise you. I confess
that I have no great feelings of praise right now.
It hurts to praise you. Despite all that,
I offer you a sacrifice of praise. Amen.

Honor the Lord

I asked the LORD for help,
and he saved me
        from all my fears.
Keep your eyes on the LORD!
You will shine like the sun
        and never blush with shame.
I was a nobody, but I prayed,
and the LORD saved me
        from all my troubles.

If you honor the LORD,
        his angel will protect you.
Discover for yourself
        that the LORD is kind.
Come to him for protection,
        and you will be glad.

> Honor the LORD!
>   You are his special people.
> No one who honors the LORD
>   will ever be in need.

— Psalm 34:4-9, CEV

Thank you, God, for setting your angel over me.
I feel your hand of protection. I am a nobody.
But I am a nobody who trusts in you. Amen.

Paralyzed

Some men came, bringing to him a paralytic, carried by four of them. Since they could not get him to Jesus because of the crowd, they made an opening in the roof above Jesus and, after digging through it, lowered the mat the paralyzed man was lying on. When Jesus saw their faith, he said to the paralytic, "Son, your sins are forgiven."

—Mark 2:3-5, NIV

"Some men came, bringing to him a paralytic." Sometimes having cancer feels like being paralyzed, not so much physically but emotionally and spiritually. I thought I was a person with a firm faith and able to cope well—until I got cancer. Suddenly my world turned topsy-turvy. Drugs and sickness blurred my ability to reason. I was confused and dazed. I tried to pray, but I couldn't concentrate.

The words in the Bible seemed like hieroglyphics. God was a puzzle. I tried to muster faith, but I felt, well . . . paralyzed.

The wonderful thing about this story is that this man was paralyzed, helpless, trapped—yet that didn't paralyze the faith of his friends. They physically and spiritually lifted him up to Jesus.

And it gets better. The Gospel says "when Jesus saw their faith," he healed the man. It doesn't say "when he saw the faith of the paralyzed man" but rather "when he saw the faith of the friends." If you feel emotionally or spiritually paralyzed, know that God has mercy on you and that God is hearing the prayers of all your friends that are being lifted on your behalf. When you are sick, it is so hard sometimes to do anything but be sick. Rest, and let others do the work of faith and intercession on your behalf.

O God, I feel so weak. It is more than I can do to even lift up a prayer to you beyond "Help!" Thank you that I am not alone—that you hear the prayers of my brothers and sisters in the faith that are going up on my behalf. Amen.

Life Will Return

It's not a sure thing, but people often do survive cancer. This author did. Twice. And, believe it or not, life can return to normal. I know that there were times when I could not see surviving as an alternative. I could see more and harsher treatments and I could see dying, but I lost consciousness of the possibility of more and good regular life.

Focus on that now. Think of something that you loved to do before cancer, and see yourself doing it again. Daydream for a minute. See yourself doing it again in the future. Make it a goal.

Some friends helped me with this. They bought me tennis balls and a volleyball net in the middle of some rough treatments. Or think of something that you would love to do. It might be to pig out on a delicious meal of your favorite dishes without any thought to your current, restrictive diet. It might be a trip to Florida or Cancún or skiing in Taos. It might be that special thing you always wanted to do but never seemed to be able to break away and do. Put it in your future. Make it a reward. Just two more of these awful treatments and I get to . . .

> *O Lord, life has so many pleasant possibilities.*
> *I have lost sight of them in my suffering.*
> *I remember all the good gifts that are a part*
> *of ordinary living. I look forward to enjoying*
> *some more of your earthly delights. Amen.*

When God Says No

Three times I begged the Lord to make
this suffering go away. But he replied,
"My kindness is all you need. My power
is strongest when you are weak." So if
Christ keeps giving me his power, I will
gladly brag about how weak
I am. Yes, I am glad to be weak or
insulted or mistreated or to have troubles and sufferings, if it is for Christ.
Because when I am weak,
I am strong.
                    —2 Corinthians 12:8-10, CEV

An amazing thing comes to light when we look at
the times when God said no to people's prayer
requests. God said no to some of whom we would
consider the most spiritual people in the Bible.
When his baby was dying, King David asked God
to spare the child's life. God said no. The apostle

Paul asked God to take away an illness so that he might preach the gospel better. God said no. Our Savior Jesus asked God if there was any way he could forgo the cross. God said no.

In none of these situations, however, did God's no cause these people to lose faith. They trusted that God was doing the thing that was the best for all concerned. Their faith was based on more than what they could get out of God. They let God have the job of being God. They didn't second-guess God's decisions.

Master, help me to remember that no is a real answer from a loving God. Your no comes out of a heavenly perspective. It comes straight out of your great love for me. Amen.

God, My Protector

In times of trouble,
    you will protect me.
You will hide me in your tent
and keep me safe
    on top of a mighty rock.
You will let me defeat
    all of my enemies.
Then I will celebrate,
    as I enter your tent
with animal sacrifices
    and songs of praise.

Please listen when I pray!
    Have pity. Answer my prayer.
My heart tells me to pray.
I am eager to see your face,
    so don't hide from me.
I am your servant,
and you have helped me.

—Psalm 27:5-9, CEV

Where could I turn, except to you, O God?
You know me. You have promised
that you are committed to the best for me.
I don't always know what the best for me is,
but I know where to go to get love. Amen.

Worse Than Dying

I was watching a television interview one day, and the person being interviewed said something that shocked me. He was a terminal cancer patient, and the interviewer had asked him, "Are you afraid to die?" At that time in my life, my answer would have been, "Yes! Yes! A thousand times yes!"

But the man replied, "There are worse things than dying." "Worse things than dying," I thought. "You've got to be kidding me!" But the more I thought about it, the more I realized that he was right. After all, we have to die sometime, even if we live to 120. So there's only prolonging life and postponing death.

The question comes down to what we are going to do with however many years we do have. What is worse than dying? To be alive but to not really live. To not know and share love. To not make something worthwhile out of your existence. To have not figured out why you're here. To have never shared a sandwich with a friend. To have never really seen the sky. To never have given of yourself to someone in need. To never have met your loving Maker. Yes, there are things that are worse than dying.

O God, let me live and honor you
while I am alive. Let me enter into your presence
knowing that I have used this gift of life well.
Help me to live to your glory today. Amen.

Not Dead Yet

A Monty Python movie has a poor soul dragged before the supposed Spanish Inquisition. After he refuses to repent of his ways, the judges decide to be done with him. They pummel him, then turn to leave. But he calls up to them, "I'm not dead yet!" So they pummel him some more, kicking, punching, hitting. Again they turn to leave, but he croaks, "I'm not dead yet!"

This ridiculous scene repeats itself several times. Goofy, yes. But I've found strength in those words: "I'm not dead yet!" There's pluck in those words. They are the words of a gritty survivor. "Go ahead, throw at me surgeries, sleepless nights, chemotherapy, nausea, anxiety, sores, baldness, radiation burns, diarrhea, weight loss, needles, and whatever else you can think of, but I'm not dead yet! It's been hard, harder than I thought I could stand. But I did stand it. The last year or two or three have been living nightmares, but I'm not dead yet. I'm still going."

The will to live is incredible. Life can be fragile, but it can also be nearly indestructible. Look at the wars and the famines and the concentration camps, and you will see people who are survivors. What they have suffered makes the world shudder, but they came out alive and picked up life again.

I have often visited older people at hospitals and given up any hope of their recovery. I have told friends, "So and so is a goner." But they have often proved me wrong. Sometimes I visit them several years later, and they sit with a Cheshire-cat grin as if to say, "I'm not dead yet." Go ahead; be a fighter; be a survivor. Make that your little gritty motto: "I'm not dead yet!"

God of strength, help me to meet the trials of this day.
You are my power. Help me, like David, to fight
the giants around me. Amen.

Productive

We all like to feel productive, that we are doing our part, that we have contributed something. Blaise Pascal wrote, "Nothing is so intolerable to man as being fully at rest, without passion, without business, without entertainment, without care. It is then that he recognizes that he is empty, insufficient, dependent, ineffectual. From the depths of his soul now comes at once boredom, gloom, sorrow, chagrin, resentment and despair."

When we are ill for prolonged periods, we can feel useless, wondering what good we are doing still taking up space and oxygen. To be productive is a gift. Even when God created Adam and placed him in Paradise, God gave Adam a job of tending the garden.

But we are more than our ability to do. Our loved ones do not love us the less when we are disabled. A baby is still precious in its helplessness. An elderly parent still beloved. It is all right just to be today, to say, "My only goal today is to survive one more day."

There will come days when there is more than that. Perhaps there will be a remission, a cure, even a miracle. Give yourself permission to live one more day for that possibility.

> *Father, thank you that you love me for who I am,*
> *not for what I do. Thank you for today.*
> *I will live it to your glory. I wait in hope. Amen.*

God, My Shield

I love you, LORD God,
  and you make me strong.
You are my mighty rock,
  my fortress, my protector,
the rock where I am safe,
my shield, my powerful weapon,
  and my place of shelter.

I praise you, LORD!
I prayed, and you rescued me
  from my enemies.
Death had wrapped
  its ropes around me,
and I was almost swallowed
  by its flooding waters.

Ropes from the world
of the dead
  had coiled around me,

and death had set a trap
    in my path.
I was in terrible trouble
    when I called out to you,
but from your temple
you heard me
    and answered my prayer.

—Psalm 18:1 6, CEV

I know where to run when I'm in trouble, God:
straight into your arms. Hold me tight
through this frightening time. Amen.

Humor

If you are cheerful,
>   you feel good;
if you are sad,
>   you hurt all over.
—Proverbs 17:22, CEV

Go out of your way to put humor into your life.
I know you don't much feel like laughing, but
laughing is healing to your body and mind. When
you laugh chemicals are released in your brain that
strengthen your immune system and prevent
depression.

So read the funnies. Rent the Jerry Lewis video
library. Check out some Bill Cosby tapes. Buy an
elephant joke book. Read, watch, and listen to
these even when you don't feel like it. And when
you do have some spunk in you—do something
fun! Spend time with people you enjoy.

Every time I felt up to it, a friend would take me
out and play basketball with me. I was bald, shaky,

and had no reflexes, but I still enjoyed playing H-O-R-S-E and one-on-one. Tell people you have doctor's orders to take the day off and go laugh!

Loving Lord, sometimes your gifts are so simple
that we overlook them. You have given us
the ability to release healing power within ourselves.
Teach us the treasure of joy. Amen.

Rebirth

In *Peace, Love, and Healing,* Dr. Bernie Siegel talks about the immense importance of having love and hope in our lives. He notes that most of us as children did not grow up with sufficient love and hope. He suggests using our current crisis to grow on an inward level into a mature human being. Dr. Siegel writes, "It is time to move beyond that legacy of lovelessness, to forgive and be reborn. The energy for this rebirth often comes when we see and accept our own mortality" (3).

For me, cancer brought to the surface my fears, my sense of loneliness, and my own lack of peace with the universe and with God. Cancer allowed the beginning of a transformation process whose first step was to realize that I was cosmically lonely—when I reached out to the universe, I did not sense the hand of God reaching back to hold and comfort, even though it was there.

That was a hard truth to come to, but one that cancer would not allow me to ignore or deny. It forced me to see that though I said I believed in God, in reality I had been seeking from people and from the pleasures and pursuits of this world what only God can supply—peace. Cancer drove me to God, which allowed me to accept my mortality and to forgive others for not being able to fully supply what I needed most.

Lord of light, pull away all the false supports
that I have been leaning on. Show me
the empty places where I seek for peace.
Lead me on until I lean entirely on you. Amen.

Letting Go

Sometimes the pain, anxiety, sleeplessness, and confusion can be more than we can bear. A side effect of one of the steroids I was on was psychosis. With each day's pills I could feel myself creeping nearer and nearer to a mental and emotional collapse. My doctor was slow in responding to my distress signals. One day I found myself unable to hold it together anymore.

With horror I felt sensations and images and emotions that I could not control. Reeling, I asked my wife to drive me to the emergency room, and I was admitted to the psychiatric unit. The psychiatrist was sympathetic and said that this was not an unusual occurrence for people on chemotherapy. But for several days I had the unpleasant experience of feeling as if I were falling through an emotional bottomless pit—as if I were drowning and could see myself drowning but could do nothing about it. I tried so hard to keep it all together and pray and trust God, but in defeat and despair I felt myself letting go. In total weakness I let go of every rope I had lassoed God with.

But I had the wonderful experience of discovering that God did not let go of me. God had some ropes of his own, cords of compassion. Very soon into my stay at the hospital, the Spirit began to speak tenderly to me, saying, "I will never leave you or forsake you." I had the joy of finding that my relationship with God did not all depend on me.

Praise you, God, that you are committed
to holding on to me, that I do not always
have to be strong, that you will not easily
toss me aside. Like a loving parent,
you care more as I become weaker. Amen.

God Changes Everything

Here is a message for all
who are weak, trembling,
       and worried:
"Cheer up! Don't be afraid.
Your God is coming
       to punish your enemies.
God will take revenge on them
       and rescue you."

The blind will see,
and the ears of the deaf
       will be healed.
Those who were lame
       will leap around like deer;
tongues once silent
       will begin to shout.
Water will rush
       through the desert.

Scorching sand
     will turn into a lake,
and thirsty ground
     will flow with fountains.

—Isaiah 35:3-7, CEV

God, my deliverer, your promises have weight.
They can be leaned on and not give way.
You yourself stand behind them. When you speak,
it can be counted on to happen. Amen.

Joy Is a Choice

Pain is inevitable, but misery is optional. We cannot avoid pain, but we can avoid joy. God has given us such immense freedom that he will allow us to be as miserable as we want to be.

I know some people who spend their entire lives practicing being unhappy, diligently pursuing joylessness. They get more mileage from having people feel sorry for them than from choosing to live out their lives in the context of joy.

Joy is simple (not to be confused with easy). At any moment in life we have at least two options, and one of them is to choose an attitude of gratitude, a posture of grace, a commitment to joy.

There is no question that life is difficult. In fact, it has been said that God promises four things: peace, power, purpose, and TROUBLE. For example, in John 16:33 Jesus reminds us quite boldly that in the world there will be trouble. There will be tribulation, but we are not merely to endure it but to "be of good cheer," for he has overcome the world.

Many of us have only gotten half the message. We recognize the difficulty of life and drearily drag ourselves through each day, mumbling about our burdens. . . . It can be different—but the choice is ours.

—*You Gotta Keep Dancin'* by Tim Hansel

Light of the world, I choose to live in you.
I choose to believe that I am a part of something
so fantastic that eye has not seen and ear has not heard.
I joyfully get lost in the author of life. Amen.

Beauty

Seek beauty. Stop and take in the girth and the strength and the majesty of an oak. Let a flower flirt at you with a dainty blush. Get lost in a hauntingly lovely piece of music. Eat the sky with your eyes. Sit by the seashore. Breathe in the mountains. Watch children at play.

There is healing in beauty. Beauty is like a pine branch that a mountain man uses to cover his tracks—it covers over the paths of pain in your mind. The electrical pathways of our brains can be used in some areas so much that they become ruts. Experiencing the beauty of creation causes our minds to walk new paths.

Beauty flows forth from the soul of God. In the beginning God created all things beautiful. They bore an image of their Creator. God's scent—a sense of the Spirit having passed close by—is present both in the natural world around us and in humans when we reflect God's being in our living and creating. It is like walking through an artist's studio, seeing his or her work all around you. You feel in some sense that the artist is present. When we inhale the fragrance of a flower, we are touching and being touched by its Creator. God soothes us with the beauty that flows from his inward being.

Master Artist, all that your hand touches
reflects your beauty. Heal the pain and sorrow.
Touch me, and make me whole.
I soak in your presence. Amen.

Fear of Dying

Would you think ill of me if I told you that even when I became a minister, I still had a pretty healthy fear of dying? The longer that I've lived, the less afraid I have become. But there's still a little bit of fear there. It's not fear of judgment. It's the fear of the unknown.

Some people in life are adventuresome. They love to see what's just around the corner. They live for the excitement of the new. Then there are the people like me. People who are just fine with what they have and where they are. We enjoy a sense of security. We would rather have the one so-so life in the hand than trade it for the heavenly two in the bush.

The Lord helped me see the ridiculousness of this fear when I was a young boy. My parents came to me and told me that it was time to move. I didn't want to move. I was quite happy where I was. I had everything I needed. My parents promised me that I would be going to an exciting place, that I would make friends, that it would be so much better than I could imagine. I wouldn't budge. It got so bad that the doctor had to use forceps to get me out!

Yes, I am talking about being born. You see, we've all already done this once in our existence—moved from one relatively happy environment to one so much more than we could have conceived of. Just imagine, when you were in your mother's womb, if someone had tried to tell you that just three inches away was a whole world of color and sound and relationships and space beyond your wildest imagination. Think of this world as a second womb, and you may be about to be born into heaven. Don't make the doctor use forceps!

Whether you survive cancer or not, let go of the fear.

Our Father in heaven, give me a heart
that does not fear the future that you
are preparing for me. I confess my own anxiety.
Create in me a sense of expectancy. Amen.

Only God Knows

Where then is wisdom?
It is hidden from human eyes
        and even from birds.
Death and destruction
have merely heard rumors
        about where it is found.
God is the only one who knows
        the way to wisdom,
because he sees everything
        beneath the heavens.
When God divided out
        the wind and the water,
and when he decided the path
        for rain and lightning,
he also determined the truth
        and defined wisdom.
God told us, "Wisdom means
that you respect me, the Lord,
        and turn from sin."

—Job 28:20-28, CEV

Almighty Creator, I confess that this world confuses me.
Sometimes you confuse me, too.
Without fully understanding, I trust, I submit.
Who else is there but you?
I would be a fool not to trust you. Amen.

The Privilege of Trusting

Sometimes it helps to back up and view something from a radically different perspective. Instead of concentrating on how hard it is when it feels like God isn't there, focus on the opportunity that God is giving you. Say out loud, "God is giving me the privilege of trusting in his Word in the absence of experience."

Does that sound crazy to you? Consider the words of Jesus. In the Gospel of John the disciple Thomas refuses to believe that Jesus has risen from the dead without absolute, empirical evidence: "Unless I see the nail marks in his hands and put my finger where the nails were, and put my hand into his side, I will not believe it."

Jesus appears to him and invites him to touch and see. Then he says a remarkable thing: "Because you have seen me, you have believed; blessed are those who have not seen and yet have believed" (John

20:25,29, NIV). Blessed are those who believe in his Word in the absence of experience! Why?

To believe without seeing is a sign of respect to the one who has promised. My wife and I sold a car, and the man wanted to write a check. "I'm good for it," he said. We had a choice—to trust the man's word or to demand cash. Though we considered asking for cash, we chose to pay the man the compliment that we believed that he was a man of character. Can we pay God that same compliment? The Lord is offering us the privilege.

Master, thank you for the privilege
you are offering me to pay you a compliment.
I choose to trust you in spite
of all the conditions and feelings
telling me not to. I choose to give you glory
over my own needs. Amen.

All We Need
to Know

Anyone who suffers wrestles with the question why. And anyone who wrestles with that question long enough and seriously enough comes to the conclusion that on this earth we will never comprehend an adequate answer. The Bible gives hints and clues. We see various good results that come from suffering, such as patience and endurance and a witness to others. But God is forthright about the fact that we are not able to fully understand God's ways. "Just as the heavens are higher than the earth, my thoughts and my ways are higher than yours" (Isaiah 55:9, CEV).

Where does that leave us as people caught in the need to know why we are going through what we are going through? This question frustrated and debilitated me all through my first bout with cancer and beyond.

Finally the Spirit of God spoke to me. "Either I am, or I am not; those are your only two choices."

Try as I may, I could not not believe in God. That left this whole universe a giant, meaningless accident. Impossible—and hopeless. Then the second message came. "Either Jesus is the express image of my nature, or he is a charlatan." Jesus, a charlatan? The man who spoke the most wise and penetrating words ever? The glory of the one who hung upon the cross carrying the sins of the world? A charlatan? Impossible. The final part of the message came. "Then if I am, and if Jesus is my incarnation, then I must be a God who loves you infinitely. That is all you ever need to know."

O God, I do believe in you—it is impossible
not to. And I do believe in your Son—
my precious Savior, Jesus. Looking at divine love
hanging on the cross is all I ever need to know. Amen.

Why Me?

Sometimes the question is asked, "Why does God allow pain and suffering?" I defer that question to God. But another question is easier to answer: "Why me?"

The answer is simple. "Why not you?" I am not trying to be hard, but nowhere does the Bible say that either humans in general or Christians specifically are exempt from trials and suffering. The book of Genesis tells us that as a result of the sin of Adam and Eve, all of humanity—even the earth itself—is under a curse. Hardship, pain, suffering, and death were all released. God put Adam and Eve outside of the garden of perfection and put angelic guards to keep them out.

In compassion, God sent Jesus to begin to reverse the curse. But the finality of that reversal comes only at the end of time. There is no promise to Christians that once they accept Christ, they will never have to work by the sweat of the brow or have pain in childbirth or get cancer or die. Listen to the litany of sufferings of the apostle Paul:

> I have worked much harder, been in prison more frequently, been flogged more severely, and been exposed to death again and again. Five times I received from the Jews the forty lashes minus one. Three times I was beaten with rods, once I was stoned, three times I was shipwrecked, I spent a night and a day in the open sea, I have been constantly on the move. . . . I have labored and toiled and have often gone without sleep; I have known hunger and thirst and have often gone without food; I have been cold and naked.
> —2 Corinthians 11:23-27, NIV

The only promise that we have as Christians is the promise of Jesus, "And surely I am with you always, to the very end of the age" (Matthew 28:20, NIV). Even Jesus suffered and died, then entered into paradise. Why you? Why not you?

O Lord, I hurt. Give me the comfort that you gave to Paul and to your Son. I thank you that you are giving me the strength to bear up under the pressure. Amen.

Your Love

Your love is faithful, Lord,
and even the clouds in the sky
        can depend on you.
Your decisions are always fair.
They are firm like mountains,
        deep like the sea,
and all the people and animals
        are under your care.

Your love is a treasure,
and everyone finds shelter
        in the shadow of your wings.
You give your guests a feast
        in your house,
and you serve a tasty drink
        that flows like a river.
The life-giving fountain
        belongs to you,
and your light gives light
        to each of us.

—Psalm 36:5-9, CEV

If I weren't upheld by your love, God,
I would surely be in a mess.
I don't know how people make it
if they don't have you to lean on.
This cancer is not easy, but your love keeps me
from drowning. Amen.

Sadness

On this earth we don't have a city
that lasts forever, but we are waiting
for such a city.

—Hebrews 13:14, CEV

I found that cancer put me in touch with the sadness of the world. After I got cancer, everywhere I looked was someone suffering. Cancer released a sympathy that was almost overwhelming. I struggled with this because it seemed that everyone said that a Christian should be joyous all of the time.

Through time I began to come to a balance. The joy comes from God—the knowledge that God is there and that God cares. But there is a place for sorrow, too. It is a sorrow that I believe lives in the heart of God as well—the sorrow of a world reaping the results of living outside of God's perfect will.

God did not design the world with suffering, sorrow, or death in mind. These are the second best that we chose for ourselves. We are living in a second-best world. God has promised to take us to a first-class world someday. Until then, there is good reason for sadness. Sadness is a mark of maturity. It is the trait of someone who is home-sick, who knows and longs for a better place.

The lie is pervasive that if we work hard, we can make this world feel like home. It is not home. Cancer reminds us of that.

O God, I weep with you over a creation
that chose second best. I know that with this cancer
I am not experiencing your perfect will for me. I long
for that enduring city that is my real home. Amen.

Depression

> Elijah was afraid when he got her
> message, and he ran to the town of
> Beersheba in Judah. He left his servant
> there, then walked another whole day
> into the desert. Finally, he came to
> a large bush and sat down in its shade.
> He begged the LORD, "I've had enough.
> Just let me die! I'm no better off than
> my ancestors." Then he lay down in the
> shade and fell asleep.
>
> —1 Kings 19:3-5, CEV

Of all of the surgeries, procedures, and treatments that I was put through, I can say with confidence that the most painful thing I experienced was not physical—it was depression. Depression can come from the rough times that we go through and the possibility of death. But, as cancer patients, we get steroids and drugs that can chemically alter our minds and induce depression. The black thoughts and oppressive clouds of despair that follow us around are often harder to deal with than simple physical pain.

Depression is a hidden disease. Many people are ashamed of it. But statistics show that 39 percent of all people experience clinical depression sometime in life—and that is without having chemotherapy drugs to help them along! Whatever its source, depression results in our brains getting chemically off balance. In the last few decades treatment of depression has shifted more and more away from psychotherapy or counseling to medicating in order to restore that balance. Nonaddictive antidepressants can help us get back to a healthy emotional state.

Even such spiritual greats as Elijah experienced the trauma of depression. God treated him as the spiritual/psychological/physical creature that we all are. God gave him food and drink, rest, and a gentle whisper to his soul.

O Lord, the darkness is great, and I cannot see my way. I reach out for you through the mists of gloom. I know that you can see me even when I cannot see you. Amen.

No Magic Formulas

Sometimes, no matter what we may wish, try, or pray for, we are left with what we are—depressed. There are no magic formulas, no snapping of fingers, and, though miracles do occasionally happen, they don't seem to be the norm. To be sure, try all the easy fixes—pray, think cheerful thoughts, take medication. Still, sometimes we just have to slough it through.

I went to a Christian psychiatrist to get his wisdom. I said, "Doc, I'm really depressed." He said, "No wonder, look what you're going through. I'd be depressed, too!" That didn't fix anything, but it was a good reality check. You've got cancer— that's *hard!*

Most people will understand. A few won't. Because they have never had real depression, they will try to tell you to quit moping and be happy. They will drive you crazy!

Read the book of Job. Read the psalms. They are not filled with pat answers and easy fixes. They are filled with moaning and groaning and "how long-ing?" It's amazing how candid the Bible is about the fact that sometimes life is hard. There is no attempt to whitewash things and say, "If you just believe in God, everything will come up daisies."

Are you depressed? That's hard—but it's all right. I can assure you, I got depressed each time I had cancer.

O God, there is no comfort where I am. It is hard.
I need relief. I will keep calling out to you until you
bring me out of this trial. Amen.

The Lord Rescues

Descendants of Jacob,
I, the LORD, created you
    and formed your nation.
Israel, don't be afraid.
    I have rescued you.
I have called you by name;
    now you belong to me.
When you cross deep rivers,
I will be with you,
    and you won't drown.
When you walk through fire,
you won't be burned
    or scorched by the flames.

I am the LORD, your God,
the Holy One of Israel,
    the God who saves you.
I gave up Egypt, Ethiopia,
and the region of Seba
    in exchange for you.

To me, you are very dear,
and I love you.
That's why I gave up nations
and people to rescue you.

—Isaiah 43:1-4, CEV

You love me—that's all I need to know, Lord.
I am walking through the fire of cancer.
In you, I will emerge without even the smell
of smoke upon me. I will not be afraid. Amen.

Tired of Surviving

I was talking to one of my parishioners. She has a rare cancer that her doctors call incurable. For two years she has fought valiantly for life. The physicians have tried extremely harsh and experimental treatments to keep her alive. They hold out a slim hope of winning out against stacked odds. Every day of life holds out the possibility of a new medical breakthrough. If nothing else, she has eked out two more years of life.

But on the phone she confessed to me, "I don't know how much longer I can do this. If this experimental treatment doesn't work, how can I explain to my family that I don't want to try any more? I am too tired to keep on fighting."

Is it wrong to give up? Does God want us to scratch for every last ounce of painful life? I am not talking about suicide. The Bible never presents suicide as a faithful option. But in our age of advanced medical treatment and technology, the question surfaces, "Do I have to use every possible option to stay alive?"

I believe there are times when the answer is no. If you are listening for the voice of God, and the Spirit is saying to you, "Don't give up. Have courage. Keep going. You have responsibilities. I am not finished with you yet," then by all means obey. But our society has become guilty of not always believing what we confess. We say that heaven is a much better place, but we act as if we must avoid going there like the plague. We act as if dying and going to heaven are the most awful things we can think of. Often we make life on earth an idol. Sometimes it is a lack of faith that keeps us trying past the point of reasonableness. If you are struggling with this issue, go to God and get the Great Physician's opinion.

God, I'm listening. Forgive me if I have accidentally
slipped into not believing your Word.
If you want me to keep fighting, give me courage.
If my fight is done, give me peace. Amen.

Forgive

"And when you stand praying, if you
hold anything against anyone, forgive
him, so that your Father in heaven may
forgive you your sins."
                              —Mark 11:25, niv

A lot of times cancer involves someone, somewhere, doing something stupid or irresponsible.
Maybe you are a smoker and got lung cancer, or you
spent too much time sunbathing and got skin
cancer. The first time I had cancer I went to the
doctor about some suspicious lumps. She laughed
and said they were nothing. By the time I got the
nerve to mention them to her again, I was in the
final stages of Hodgkin's disease. Or maybe you are
one of those people who experience symptoms for
months and ignore them, stubbornly resisting the
trip to the doctor.

Two words are needed: forgive and change. What has happened has happened. In the mystery of life, it was ordained that cancer be a part of your experience. Forgive anyone and everyone responsible. Unforgiveness blocks the peace of God. Joseph had just cause to hold a grudge against his brothers. But he said to them, "You intended to harm me, but God intended it for good" (Genesis 50:20, NIV).

At the same time, if there are changes that need to be made, make them. Get a new doctor. Stop smoking. Pay attention to what your body is telling you. You cannot change the past, but you can learn from it to guide your future.

Lord, I forgive anyone who did me harm,
myself included. I am here for a reason
and a purpose. Let me cut the anchor
of bitterness and set the sail of experience. Amen.

Pride and Humility

Twelve months later, as the king was walking on the roof of the royal palace of Babylon, he said, "Is not this the great Babylon I have built as the royal residence, by my mighty power and for the glory of my majesty?"

The words were still on his lips when a voice came from heaven, "This is what is decreed for you, King Nebuchadnezzar: Your royal authority has been taken from you. You will be driven away from people and will live with the wild animals; you will eat grass like cattle. Seven times will pass by for you until you acknowledge that the Most High is sovereign over the kingdoms of men and gives them to anyone he wishes."

—Daniel 4:29-32, NIV

God sent upon Nebuchadnezzar a debilitating condition to tame his pride. Nebuchadnezzar came to see that all that he had and was came from God. I doubt that most of our cancers are a rebuke to our exalted egos. Nonetheless, cancer does have a way of stripping away all of our feelings of self-sufficiency.

Our ability to earn a living is threatened. Our mental clarity diminishes. Strength dries up like a baked mud puddle. We can barely take care of ourselves or maybe not at all. We become extremely aware that the essence of our life is in the hand of someone greater than we are.

Let us use our cancer as an opportunity to humble our spirits before the throne and give the rightful glory due to God.

God of glory, my existence flows from the source of your being. Forgive me for the times I ever thought I was running the universe. I place myself in the hands of the One greater than I. Amen.

New Heaven and New Earth

I saw a new heaven and a new earth.
The first heaven and the first earth
     had disappeared, and so had the sea.
Then I saw New Jerusalem, that holy city,
     coming down from God in heaven.
It was like a bride dressed in her wedding gown
and ready to meet her husband.

I heard a loud voice shout from the throne:
     God's home is now with his people.
     He will live with them, and they will be
          his own.
     Yes, God will make his home among
          his people.

He will wipe away all tears from their eyes,
and there will be no more
death, suffering, crying, or pain.
These things of the past are gone
forever.

—Revelation 21:1-4, CEV

Lord, you have given me life. For the most part
it has been good. Help me to trust that you
are preparing something much better.
I will enjoy this life while I have it, but I wait
in anticipation for that place beyond compare. Amen.

Escape

Finally, [Elijah] came to a large bush and
sat down in its shade. He begged the
Lord, "I've had enough. Just let me die!"
—1 Kings 19:4, CEV

Judas threw the money into the temple
and then went out and hanged himself.
—Matthew 27:5, CEV

When a person is in a difficult situation, the natural thing to do is to review all of the possible ways
out of that situation. Some of the possibilities may
be outside of God's laws. They become possibilities that we choose to bypass out of obedience to
God. Then we take the best path out of the
remaining choices.

If you need a car in order to go to work but you're
short on money, you could get a loan, walk, rob
somebody, beg, buy a lottery ticket, pray for a miracle, get a job closer to home, move closer to work,

carpool, or ride the bus. Some of these options you're not going to take because, although they are perhaps the easiest and quickest ways, they are obviously displeasing to God. Once they are eliminated, you begin to pray to discern the best choice or choices that God has for you.

When we're in deep pain and frightening circumstances, it is only natural that one of the options that comes to us is to prematurely end our lives. Suicide seems to have occurred to Elijah, and many times it ran through my mind as a possibility. But I saw it for what it was—a suggestion that came out of my natural man, one that should be rejected because it does not bring glory to God.

It is not wrong to have the thought of suicide come to our minds, but it is sin to act on it, as Judas did.

God, I turn to you to supply my needs.
Give me strength to endure what I must endure
to be faithful to you. I look to you for my rescue. Amen.

Still Afraid

What were your expectations when the doctors pronounced you cancer-free? Did you expect to dance with joy, eat a steak dinner, and resume life where you left off? Some people can do that, but for many people a new set of realities can make returning to a carefree life difficult.

For one, cancer has stripped us of all our illusions of immortality. There is a new grasp of the fragility of life. Every cold, cough, tremor, fever, or irregularity makes us wonder if it is cancer-related. There is the real possibility of recurrence. For most of us, the doctor did not just release us. He or she set up an appointment to return for an exam in three or six months. Why? Because doctors can never be certain that they have killed or removed every cancer cell in our body. Checkups become for us times of life-and-death import.

Sometimes our friends do not understand. They think we should be on cloud nine. They do not realize how they would feel if every three months they were going to find out whether they have cancer or not.

There are good reasons to be afraid. We can be glad we are done while still fearing that this is only an interlude. We must learn to take our fears to God and allow the Spirit to comfort us. God spoke to Joshua's fears: "Do not be terrified; do not be discouraged, for the LORD your God will be with you wherever you go" (Joshua 1:9, NIV). Jesus added, "Do not let your hearts be troubled. Trust in God; trust also in me" (John 14:1, NIV).

God, when have I ever really been safe and secure
apart from you? My real safety comes from being held
in the palm of your hand. Remind me again that you
are in control and that you are taking care of me. Amen.

The Future

The future. What does it hold for me? Will the cancer come back? Will I have to go through chemotherapy again? Will I survive a second bout?

When I finished my treatments, I could not relax and enjoy life. All of the possibilities haunted me. My oncologist had said that as far as he could tell, the cancer was gone. "But," he warned, "you will not be out of the woods until five years have passed. Even then recurrence is possible. Something in your body went wrong in the first place to cause this cancer. It could happen again. Furthermore," as if that were not enough, "you are now more likely to develop leukemia."

How do we get back to the business of living when all these goblins hover over us? Wendy Schlessel Harpham in *After Cancer: A Guide to Your New Life* tells us that we can see the answer if we think about a six-inch-wide balancing beam. If the beam were set just a few inches off of the ground, we could all walk on it with the greatest of ease. But if it were raised five feet off of the ground, most of us would totter, wave our arms wildly, and fall. Why? Because we lose our focus on the beam and begin to focus on the ground. Gymnasts learn to refocus on the beam and not on the ground.

The Israelites also had to be taught to focus on God and the Lord's present provision rather than worry about the future. In the wilderness, when God gave them manna, the miracle bread, God would not allow them to gather any more than one day's worth at a time. God seemed to be saying, "I provided today. Tomorrow, when it is today again, I will provide again." Work on focusing on this day that God has blessed you with.

Master, help me to set my eyes on Jesus, the author and perfecter of my faith. Help me not to look down, not to look within, but to look up. Amen.

The Lord Gives Strength

Don't you know?
> Haven't you heard?
The Lord is the eternal God,
> Creator of the earth.
He never gets weary or tired;
his wisdom cannot be measured.

The Lord gives strength
> to those who are weary.
Even young people get tired,
> then stumble and fall.
But those who trust the Lord
> will find new strength.
They will be strong like eagles
> soaring upward on wings;
they will walk and run
> without getting tired.

—Isaiah 40:28-31, CEV

I am weary, O God. Give me strength.
My treatments are like a vampire
that sucks all my energy away.
I am tired of being tired.
Show me your new strength
that I may soar like an eagle. Amen.

Time to Heal

The doctor has said those magic words, "You're finished with treatment. The cancer appears to be gone." Thank God! You are given a follow-up appointment and waved out the door. Few doctors tell you this, but you are not done. The disease is gone, but the healing has just begun. Depending on the depth of your experience, you may have multiple years before your body, mind, and spirit are healed to their full capacity.

Your body feels old, depleted, and tired. Do not despair. It will get much of its old bounce back, but it may take a year or two. It will be a while before the fatigue, decreased mental clarity, extra need for sleep, and lack of appetite disappear. Don't expect to run the marathon in a month. After my last bout with cancer it took two years for there to be adequate saliva in my mouth, three years for the nerve damage in my feet to heal, and four years for my stamina to return and my immune system to recover.

Stress, anxiety, and fear don't disappear overnight, either. Time truly is a healer of wounds, but time is required. Two years after my cancer, I was sitting with some Christian friends, and I was feeling jealous of their high spirits and frustrated by my lack of enthusiasm. I prayed to God about it. The Spirit gave me a picture of a famous pro basketball player who was forced to sit on the bench for the whole season because the coach wanted him healed for the play-offs. God's words came to me, "Take time to heal. There will be plenty of work to do in the future."

God, give me patience. I thought I was done with the race, but I see there are still several more miles to run. Help me to be thankful for how far I've come. Thank you that you are still continuing to heal me inside and out. Amen.

Disabilities

Cancer often leaves us a little less than we were pre-cancer—less energy, minus an organ or two, less physically attractive, a compromised immune system, blind, a weak heart. It is easy to feel sorry for ourselves—to concentrate on our lacks.

I was having trouble in this area. It occurred to me to read Helen Keller's autobiography to see how she dealt with feeling sorry for herself due to her lacks. I discovered that she dwelled, not on her disabilities, but rather on her abilities. Perhaps it was because she was very young when she lost her hearing and her sight. Perhaps she had no real sense of what she didn't have; therefore she saw her circumstances as normal.

This brought a new thought to my mind. I do not have the ability to fly. Birds do. But I do not feel sorry for myself because I can't, nor am I jealous of birds because they can. I view my own situation as normal despite what I could view as a disability. I also do not have the keen sense of smell that my dog has. Yet, again, I do not mourn my lack. There are so many other things that I can do that I spend zero minutes a day feeling sorry for myself because I can't fly or track a rabbit. In the same way I do not grieve because I possess neither Michael Jordan's athletic prowess nor Luciano Pavarotti's voice.

Make that shift in your own mind. View what you have as what you have. It is normal for you. The only reason you are mourning is that you remember once having that ability. You, however, are a different person than you were. Now, consider what all you can do with what you have. I bet there is still a great deal left. Get out and do those things. I also bet there are things you never had time to do before because you were too busy doing other things. Like Helen Keller, see how far you can fly with the gifts and abilities that you do have.

Lord of life, show me the wide world out in front of me. I will not be jealous of dogs or birds, pro athletes or professional singers, or of the self that I was. I embark on the adventure of finding out what I am capable of doing. Amen.

Painful Prayer

For two or three years after each of my cancer experiences I found that I had trouble praying. It hurt emotionally to pray. I would try to pray but found myself unable to sustain a prolonged prayer. The problem was that, to a certain degree, I had to struggle with learning to trust God again.

Cancer often opens our eyes to the reality that God and this universe are much more mysterious and enigmatic than we had realized. Cancer showed me that I had taken my Bible and had drawn a picture of God and the world with all the loose ends tied up. The problem was not with the Bible. The problem was that I had oversimplified it.

It is a little like living with your normal, run-of-the-line father for twenty years, only to discover that he is also the top CIA operative in the world. You have to reexamine every aspect of your relationship in a new light and see if this is still a man you can believe and respect. Was that trip to Paris really just a family vacation? Did he ever put you in danger?

I had to reexamine my relationship with God and my understanding of the Bible from a new perspective to know in my innermost self that God is trustworthy, that God loves me, that God has my best interests at heart. It takes time to learn to look a more realistic picture of God in the eye and love and praise him.

God Almighty, I'm having trouble trusting you right now. You are much more awesome than I realized. Be kind to me while I struggle to come to a more mature faith. Amen.

A Prayer of Thanks

I will praise you, Lord!
      You saved me from the grave
and kept my enemies
      from celebrating my death.
I prayed to you, Lord God,
      and you healed me,
saving me from death
      and the grave.

Your faithful people, Lord,
will praise you with songs
      and honor your holy name.
Your anger lasts a little while,
but your kindness lasts
      for a lifetime.
At night we may cry,
but when morning comes
      we will celebrate.

—Psalm 30:1-5, CEV

What would I do
if I didn't have you, Lord?
Where would I go?
Who would hear me?
I celebrate that I have you
to turn to in my troubles. Amen.

Give Thanks

The Bible says that we should "give thanks in all circumstances" (1 Thessalonians 5:18, NIV). Does this include cancer? Notice it does not say we should be thankful *for* everything, rather *in* everything. Though we may not be particularly thankful for having cancer, there are many things in our cancer experience that we can be thankful for.

We can be thankful for

- The love of God that upholds us and never deserts us.
- The more mature traits, such as perseverance and a new strength of character, that develop from going through the trials.
- An intensified sense that our days on earth are numbered, that we must use our time here on earth well.
- A deepened empathy for others who are hurting, perhaps even a new ministry to those in crisis.
- The witness that our struggle has provided.

- Strengthened bonds of love for those who were there when we needed them and a clearer vision of what real love looks like.
- A new set of priorities and a realization of the unimportance of so many things.
- A deeper cherishing of life and the realization that heaven is a better place.
- The peace that comes with having looked death in the eye and seeing that it is something that Christ has conquered.
- A fuller confidence in both our own emotional strength and God's sufficient grace in our weaknesses.
- A more mature relationship with God.

God, thank you for the unasked-for bag of gifts
that cancer has provided. Thank you
that you never left me nor forsook me.
Thank you for the gift of still being alive. Amen.

At Ease

The enemy is spotted. An alarm goes off, and the entire base goes on red alert. Every eye is peeled. No one is dozing on the job. Each gunner is ready to fire in an instant.

Just like a military base, our bodies are designed to have several levels of intensity—at ease, semi-alert, and red alert. When our bodies are at red alert, we are ready for instant fight or flight. Adrenaline is flowing. Muscles are tense. Hearts race.

A prolonged and difficult cancer treatment can have the effect of causing our bodies and our psyches to get stuck in red alert. So many life-threatening situations have been thrown at us that we forget how to be at ease.

After the immediate danger of cancer has passed, we can find ourselves unable to relax and let go of the stress. Every bothersome bit of trivia in our daily life causes a full-scale scramble. A small snafu develops at work. The grocery store is closed when we need cat food. Our children miss the school bus. Friends come over when the house isn't spick-and-span. Red alert. Red alert. Red alert. Red alert.

This is an uncomfortable and wearing way to live. We need to learn how to react again at an appropriate degree to the level of the crisis. It helps to talk to ourselves. Say out loud, "Is the spilled milk really a major disaster?" No. Tell yourself that. Check with friends to confirm what your mind is telling you. Make yourself learn to stand down. Try some relaxation techniques. Perhaps you'll need some tranquilizers for a while. Ask God to give you peace. "Peace I leave with you; my peace I give you" (John 14:27, NIV).

Loving Creator, you have given our body needed responses. Help me to retrain myself. Give me your peace from heaven. Amen.

Memories

I was at a local hospital visiting one of my parishioners. After the visit, I went to the cafeteria to get
some lunch. I glanced up and out the window at
the adjoining building. I could see the very window
that I had looked out of the year before — the
room in the psychiatric unit where I had spent a
week due to side effects from steroids. A plethora
of unpleasant memories came pouring in.

Many things trigger our memories: checkups,
the anniversary of a diagnosis or a bone marrow
transplant, smells, people, holidays, and places.
Memories can produce any combination of feelings from anxiety, depression, a sense of disloca-
tion, and weepiness to overwhelming thankfulness
and joy.

If your memories cause you too much emotional
pain, then try not to wallow in them. Reliving bad
experiences can have the effect of reviving feelings
that you are not ready to deal with. These feelings
will come out some time and some place, but you

can choose to put them off until you are in a healthier emotional state to deal with them.

In the meantime, focus on reinforcing the positive and good feelings. Let your memory remind you to give thanks for your healing, for all your caring friends, and for your promising future. The apostle Paul said, "Forgetting what is behind and straining toward what is ahead, I press on" (Philippians 3:13-14, NIV).

When you are ready, relive your memories little by little in the presence of God, and allow the Lord to tenderly heal each one.

Heavenly One, there is a heavy load of hurt in my soul. Take each memory and kiss it and make it feel better. Give me a picture of you holding me each time I hurt. Amen.

Almost There

I sat on the fourth floor of the administration building and looked out on the valley that spread out before me. I had come to this beautiful campus to sign up for a class. It was a little over two years since I had finished my treatment. I was about the business of getting on with my life. For so long I had had the energy to do only what life required—now I was able to start doing some of the extra things, like taking this class, that add zest to life. But there was a problem.

There was no joy. Getting up in the morning was drudgery. My work did not excite me. I didn't seem to have the extra care that makes a marriage more than a living arrangement.

I sat in a soft chair that gave me a breathtaking view, and I quieted down and listened. I listened for the voice of God. I listened for the voice of my soul. And I heard the still small voice say, "Not there yet. There is still pain inside. Much healing has taken place. Be kind to yourself."

I looked back over my two bouts with cancer as if I was looking out over the panorama before me, and various scenes and stages came in and out of focus. Then something came to me. "Write about what you went through." That is how this book began. I wrote for me as well as for you.

The apostle Paul wrote, "Praise be to the God . . . who comforts us in all our troubles, so that we can comfort those in any trouble with the comfort we ourselves have received from God" (2 Corinthians 1:3-4, NIV). Ask God to show you how to make your suffering a blessing to others. In the process, you might discover healing as well.

Master, you have taught me to listen to your voice.
Now that I am almost well, let me not stop listening.
I dedicate this whole cancer experience to you.
Show me how to comfort others
with the comfort I have received. Amen.

Notes

Notes

Notes